i'm not the new me

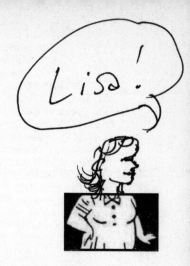

wendy mcclure

i'm not the new me

Riverhead Books
New York

Boot camp rulz!

xxoo

Wendy McClure

THE BERKLEY PUBLISHING GROUP
Published by the Penguin Group
Penguin Group (USA) Inc.
375 Hudson Street, New York, New York 10014, USA
Penguin Group (Canada), 10 Alcorn Avenue, Toronto, Ontario M4V
3B2, Canada (a division of Pearson Penguin Canada Inc.) • Penguin
Books Ltd., 80 Strand, London WC2R 0RL, England • Penguin Group
Ireland, 25 St. Stephen's Green, Dublin 2, Ireland (a division of Penguin
Books Ltd.) • Penguin Group (Australia), 250 Camberwell Road,
Camberwell, Victoria 3124, Australia (a division of Pearson Australia
Group Pty. Ltd.) • Penguin Books India Pvt. Ltd., 11 Community
Centre, Panchsheel Park, New Delhi—110 017, India • Penguin Group
(NZ), cnr Airborne and Rosedale Roads, Albany, Auckland 1310, New
Zealand (a division of Pearson New Zealand Ltd.) • Penguin Books
(South Africa) (Pty.) Ltd., 24 Sturdee Avenue, Rosebank, Johannesburg
2196, South Africa

Penguin Books Ltd., Registered Offices:
80 Strand, London WC2R 0RL, England

While this is a memoir, some events have been compressed and some
characters are composites. I have changed the names and identifying
characteristics of some of the people who appear in these pages.
Including you.

PRINTING HISTORY
First Riverhead trade paperback edition: May 2005

Library of Congress Cataloging-in-Publication Data

McClure, Wendy.
I'm not the new me / Wendy McClure.
p. cm.
ISBN 1-59448-074-5
1. McClure, Wendy. 2. Overweight women—United States—Biography.
I. Title.
RC552.O25M396 2005
362.196'398'0092—dc22
[B]   2004061480

PRINTED IN THE UNITED STATES OF AMERICA

10 9 8 7 6 5 4 3 2 1

For Mom and Dad,
and for my grandmother Vilma McClure,
with love and candy.

i'm not the new me

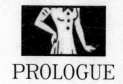

how to tell a fat girl story

You need to be brave to tell it. Very brave! You're *fat*, after all. Everybody can see that. It's assumed that your ability to recognize fat must be impaired for you to have become so damn fat in the first place. But it turns out you're *not* blind. You can cop to the truth. You're fat. How big of you to say so.

Which brings us to our next question.

You weigh how much? 173, maybe? Or 156? Or 217? 302? 195? 260? These are only suggested numbers, of course. You will have to actually *get on the scale* and see for yourself.

Don't worry. Once it has been established that You're Fat, this weighing thing is really more of a formality than anything. Because you're about to go on a journey to find yourself, to find out who you are when you're, you know, *not* fat; you're embarking on a sometimes painful odyssey through the Valley of the Shadow of Your Really Big Ass, No Offense, and it'll be a long and difficult road full of temptations and weak moments, and the territory is for the most part unmapped. So we hope you'll understand we'll just need some way to keep track of you: we'll need that number.

Oh, and you can tell us your height, if you want, but really, there's no height requirement: if you're a female and weigh more than 125 pounds, then you can have a Fat Girl Story.

So anyway. You're fat. Go on. You had to have done something to get that way.

You need to tell the world what you did. That seems like a good idea: that way, maybe people won't get fat the way you did. They'll be more vigilant the way you should have been; they won't go through life the way you did for years, paying too much attention to other things: Echo & The Bunnymen songs; your film studies papers; the light from the window eclipsing along the wall of your room.

Oh, whatever. That's not really why we're here.

We know *how* it happened. We get the "ate too much" part. Now tell us the rest. Tell us where the food came from, where you kept it, how greasy it was, or how sweet, or how much butter was involved. Don't skimp on the butter.

What else happened? What else couldn't you help eating? A Philadelphia cheese steak? Can we imagine you chewing it in slow motion and getting cheese on your face? Did it bitch-slap you, that cheese steak? And *did you love it or what?*

What about pie? Was there ever pie?

Don't be shy. Remember you're brave. You're ready to begin. In order to tell a Fat Girl Story all you need to do, for starters, is find a fat girl.

Really, it's that easy. The only catch is she can't quite be you.

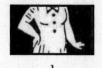

1

live and in person

I get fatter than I've ever been in my life and then I go off to Vegas for my international karaoke debut.

It happens in a place called Tong's Palace. The Chinese restaurant part of Tong's is too brightly lit and deserted; the back lounge, where we are, is dim; there are sticky tables and wobbly red chairs and strings of Christmas lights around the bar. It's four o'clock in the morning.

We're down the street from the Stratosphere hotel, where I guess there's some kind of roller coaster on the roof. We're staying at the Luxor, the hotel shaped like a big pyramid, a pyramid with a light on top that you can see from space. From *space,* so I can't possibly be trying to escape.

Though there's a moment right after I sign up to sing that I consider making a break for the bathroom or the door or the part of my head that forgets what I look like.

*   *   *

"Okay, shut *up*. You. You're?" Richard pauses here like it's a question. "Beautiful. *Okay?* And you need to know that."

The whole summer before my trip to Las Vegas, my friend Richard and I hang out at a neighborhood place we call Little Nut Hut, which is not the actual name of the establishment but rather of the dusty nut machine behind the bar and also—sometimes, depending on how pathetic I get—the nickname of the last guy I dated. Lately, I'd decided I didn't want to keep talking about him so Richard has had to come up with a new topic when we get drunk and maudlin, and to my horror it's You, Wendy, Are Fucking Fabulous, Okay? Except I don't think it's Richard's job to tell me this and I keep saying so.

"Yeah. Thanks. I'm fine." I'm mumbling. "That's not . . ." I don't want to be having this conversation again. We have it every time we're drunk. "I feel perfectly—"

"No. Shut up," he says. I do. But then I sigh a little too emphatically for him. "Shut *up!*"

"You," he says. "You deserve better. You don't even *know*. Shut up! You *don't*."

"Thanks. No. Really. I know I'm *not*, you know, ugly."

It's always sort of like an argument and I always sort of lose. Which, I think, defeats the whole point of the conversation.

Possible reasons for why I am fat: genetics; childhood issues; predisposition to depression; the Pill; Kraft Macaroni & Cheese; sedentary lifestyle; obscenely huge restaurant portions; job at bakery counter in 1985; curious grade-school diagnosis of "low blood sugar"; fears of intimacy; Western notions of Manifest Destiny; voices in my head. I mean, I don't know.

I go to the Luxor casino buffet twice, with a book. I don't usually go eat by myself like this, but some part of me has always wanted to go to one of these things alone so I wouldn't be self-conscious about how soon I'd get up to go back for more, or how many times. And I'm on a trip with a group of strangers and I need some alone time, and it's a buffet, and why not? It's tucked away somewhere on a lower level of the hotel, and thematically, it's really pretty disappointing for a place with a name like "Pharaoh's Pheast," if you must know.

I'm in Vegas because of a website. I got here through the Internet. It's a little hard to explain that to other people. You start out telling someone, "Okay, so there's this *web-site*," and that you know a few people through it, and as you're talking he or she will tilt his/her head like a dog who's heard something you can't hear, and apparently, that something is your own voice saying, *La, la, la, I have a magical pretend life*.

I should probably wonder what it is about me that makes someone think I have some deep need to escape myself. I sort of know already.

But look: I got on a plane in Chicago and came here, and I stopped in the ladies' room by the baggage claim to put on some makeup and brush my hair, and I looked in the mirror and could see myself, in my clothes. And I wear a size 22 now, and the complete strangers I came to meet will see that these are the clothes that fit me, and that I have the fucking guts to go out and buy them and put them on and appear live and in person in Las Vegas.

Though the way everyone looks here is sort of irrelevant. Everyone on this trip is—like me—a part-time writer for the website Television Without Pity, and by the time I meet them in person they are already some of the funniest people I've ever known. Seeing them is mostly a matter of adjustment: Alex is just taller than I'd imagined, Kim's quieter; Susan, more of a smoker. The truth is something you can calibrate. After a morning filled with introductions and a few hours hanging out together in one of the suites, I'm able to match faces and bodies with names; everything I know is aligned with real life, if you can call Vegas that.

The carpeting in all the casinos has patterns that are as complicated as DNA and make me feel like I'm floating. Nothing is ever quite the right size: our hotel is next door to a castle on steroids and across the street from a mini–Eiffel Tower. On our first day, a group of us wandered around the New York, New York casino and through the scaled-down replica of Greenwich Village, where some of the details are authentic enough to freak out a couple of the East Coast people. Matthew recognizes one of the building facades and he points to a set of windows above the little storefront. "Just think," he says, "in New York that's actually someone's apartment." We talked about how surreal and funny it would be to come to Las Vegas and see a midget version of your own living room window back home.

"And then, what if it wasn't just the window, but your whole apartment?" I add. We all keep discussing this: what if lavish Vegas masterminds had replicated *all* your stuff and gotten everything right—the crappy couch, the opened boxes of cereal, your cat—in three-fourths scale. That would be *fucked up*. We were laughing about it. How it would look exactly like your life until you got close to it, how then the one wrong thing would be you.

One night after we all see a movie, Pamie decides that we should do karaoke. We pile into two cabs and head out to Ellis Island, a dodgy little casino where someone told us there's karaoke at the bar. We get there just before 3 A.M. and see a couple of guys putting the microphones away; they're done for the night. They tell us about a Chinese restaurant where you can do late-night karaoke, but it's way out by the Stratosphere. We find it.

Tong's isn't crowded; we're the biggest group there. Almost everyone else there is at the bar, but we grab the big plastic binders of song lists and get a couple of tables. We take a long time studying and discussing the song lists. They have "How Am I Supposed to Live Without You" by Laura Branigan but *not* "Gloria," and what's up with that? There's a hell of a lot more Björk than one would think. But then, there are way more Blues Traveler than Bob Dylan selections. Who decides this shit? we wonder. Is there some kind of authority we can appeal to, a karaoke kourt?

Pamie gets up and sings "(You Make Me Feel Like) A Natural Woman." She's an old hand at karaoke, and her rendition is so gloriously over-the-top that everyone else loosens up. Tara sings "Killing Me Softly." Kim does "Bust a Move." Dan gets up and does an excellent and unsettling cover of "Father Figure." Everyone is shameless. I hadn't seen people perform karaoke before and I'd been under the impression that people did it to, well, show off their singing talent. Now, at Tong's, I realize what karaoke is all about: it's amateur porn for the soul.

I have trouble deciding what I'm going to perform. I can't sing very high. Or, for that matter, well. Not only do I need to find a song that's within my limited vocal range, I need to find one that I know well, by an artist who will inspire me. Prince, I decide, is perfect: a sexy little man in a ruffled shirt is just the kind of spiritual guide I need. I pick "Let's Go Crazy" from the *Purple Rain* soundtrack. I sign up and wait for my turn.

During my second visit to Pharaoh's Pheast it occurs to me that a Vegas buffet is no more about food than the casino upstairs is about money. There isn't any kind of food I particularly want here. It's the same stuff as anywhere else: macaroni, sliced turkey with gravy, vegetable medley, and dinner rolls topped with round, shiny crusts. You have some of it; you go back for more of some of it. The only thing to really wonder about is what the *more* is going to consist of.

I go all around the steam tables. I go to my seat. I watch

myself the whole time, as if I don't know what eating too much looks like. And really, I guess I don't.

I pick up the mike. "Is this on?" I say into it. Yes. Wait. No. *No,* someone's yelling from the back, so I find the switch to turn it on. I hold it and look up at a TV monitor where I can see the lyrics.

The title screen comes on. The intro starts. It's the crazy preacher part that I know by heart.

"Dearly beloved," I start. The words come on the screen: *DEARLY BELOVED.*

I am too early for *DEARLY BELOVED* and slightly too late for *WE ARE GATHERED HERE TODAY TO GET THROUGH THIS THING CALLED LIFE.* "Electric word, life, it means forever!" I scream out. "And-that's-a-mighty-long-time!" Especially when you're on a stage and you're in serious danger of messing up a Prince song and thereby and quite literally fucking up royally. "But I'm here to tell you there's something else!" I shout.

I mean, I try. This being-funny stuff is sort of new to me; I'm trying it out. Really I'm trying to get it to wear me, to fit my body around it.

"SO WHEN YOU CALL UP THAT SHRINK IN BEVERLY HILLS! YOU KNOW THE ONE! DOCTOR EVERYTHING'LL-BE-ALRIGHT . . ."

The rhythm part of the song starts. And by now the people here with me are cheering and hooting and everything is all right. I jump all around and toss my hair. I flail. I dance and dance. I don't let the elevator bring me down. I don't know what that song line means, anyway.

I learn that the red leatherette chairs at Tong's are perhaps not the most suitable things upon which to simulate the twisted, elaborate guitar solo near the end. And it seems thin air doesn't work either, at least not when you're me. But it's okay. I go crazy; I punch a higher floor.

# #

invisible jet

Dieting fat girls are always kind of like superheroes in their own fat girl stories. Of course, the fat part is the alter ego: the Clark Kent or the Diana Prince to the super-sexy spandex wonder of a woman the fat girl is one day meant to be, if she's to be anyone at all.

As superhero disguises go, fat is every bit as effective as a pair of glasses. They work on the same principle, when you think about it: the *who-would-have-thought* subterfuge. Fat girls and many kinds of incognito superheroes can transform in plain sight, moving either far too fast or too slow for the human eye to discern. But everyone is fooled once the change is complete.

Also, both fat girls and superheroes are pretty much required to have a Story of Origin. It's about the moment one realizes she looks different from everyone else, or that she's born of an alien race. Or about how she was normal once but then a laboratory accident or a broken home or a sudden genetic mutation or a summer job at Donutland changed *everything*. There's always a cause, and a fat girl is the walking, talking effect.

A fat girl story, then, ought to tell us all these things as well as describe any special powers she may possess, such as an amazing talent for making things (i.e., snacks!) disappear, or the ability to refrain from poking her own eye out whenever popular media refer to Jennifer Lopez as "plus-sized," or the power to be invisible from herself for weeks and even months at a time.

the big time

There are pictures from that night in Vegas. It is difficult not to notice that I am in some of them.

In one I am holding the microphone and looking up at the karaoke monitor. I am not facing the camera and not quite facing the side. I guess I'm in three-quarter profile only I'm showing quarters I didn't even really know I had.

But then I *do* know a lot of these parts: here is the way the fabric of my shirt comes over my hip on the side; here's how it curves under my breasts. Here is my upper chest and here is my chin, and I understand there is an additional body part that is supposed to *connect* these two things but apparently, I had only a hypothetical knowledge of my neck because *holy shit, it's fat.* Just past my jawline is a total free-for-all. It's in all the other pictures, flapping around, hanging down like dough, like the Pillsbury Dough Boy's entire and eminently pokeable pasty poofy torso only it's my *neck*, or lack thereof.

I looked at the rest of my body in the pictures and saw how my mirror had been getting it wrong all this time. All my little flabby parts added up to a whole that is much larger and far more demented than I'd allowed myself to imagine. I'd been doing the visual math wrong and the photos were like an IRS audit of my crappy accounting. They were exactly that much fun to look at.

I had a scale at home that I didn't use anymore. I hadn't used it for more than a year, in fact. It was a plain white square thing that displayed results in numerals. It never was very reliable. When I stood on it it spat out a wild range of numbers: *203! 36 . . . 140. 278!* Blink-blink. *4. 322! 231 . . . 219.* The scale language it spoke seemed to be severely impaired by some sort of Tourette's syndrome, compelled to blurt out horrible numbers before it could tell me what I really weighed. I would stand there politely and wait while it twitched and fluttered its digital eyelids. *Fat whore!* it seemed to sputter at me. *Bitch! Big-ass bitch!* I knew it didn't really mean it. But in time it became even less accurate and would just blink obscenities at me, and I'd put the stupid, broken thing away.

If I even knew how much I weighed now my mind wouldn't hold the exact number for more than an instant.

Everyone from the Vegas trip was emailing me the pictures. A few of them had web space to post photos and they'd send me links that would take me to galleries full of photos from the Saturday night dinner, the excursion to the Bellagio, the karaoke night.

When I'd sit at the computer and click on the thumbnail images there'd be two or three seconds during which the mouse-click sparked the code that sought the data to conjure up the bigger picture. It could take as long as a deep breath to happen.

You can tell my dancing is completely out of control. In one photo my head is thrown back so far it looks like I am doing the limbo. Another catches my arms in spastic chest-level chicken-wing contortions. I look like, well, like I have *special needs*.

The summer after I started college I lived in a house with three guys, one of them my best friend, Michael. We spent three months doing stupid funny stuff: we'd walk on the keys of the shitty piano that was next to the stairs; we replaced the messages in fortune cookies with ones we'd typed ourselves saying things like YOU WILL LOSE YOUR LEGS IN THE NEXT YEAR and gave them to our housemate Eric; one time Michael set off a bottle rocket in my room. Or we'd just sit around on the mattress that served as a living room couch throwing cereal at each other. We were poor but sugar was cheap and some afternoons we adapted a little too well to these conditions.

"Do that again," Michael would say, while we were trying to do something like think up dirty songs about all our friends sung to the tune of TV show themes.

"Do what again?"

"That thing with your arms," he said. "Just now, you were dancing and you looked totally retarded."

"This?" I motioned with my arms. Michael fell over laughing. I couldn't tell what was so funny.

He called in our housemate Craig. "Show Craig your tardo girl act," he said. "Come *on.*"

It seemed I could be funny without even trying and I could think of only one reason why. Only it was the thing I never let myself think about.

It was 1990 and I wore long flannel shirts, stretched-out sweaters, and lots of black. I did what I could to keep from upstaging myself.

Really, these karaoke pictures are funny. You can't tell how I sang or hear what I yelled or see my dance from one move to the next but the photos are funny as hell. They are fucking hilarious, but they catch me doing the one thing I'd never intended. They record a moment I can't get out of.

I saw two signs that read HUGE GARAGE SALE on my way back from the grocery store. It was a Saturday morning, two weeks after I'd come back from Las Vegas. I went down an alley and found the sale: a couple of chipped dining chairs, a table of odds and ends, boxes full of joyless books like *Readings in Ecology* and Maya Angelou poems. There was also a rack full of clothes, most of them hanging sweaters, though it was August. Sometimes you go to a garage sale and pick up nothing but the psychic residue from everything you see and touch there. This felt like one of those times.

There was a cassette boom box; a cheeseboard; there were old software manuals; there was a bathroom scale selling for seven dollars. One of the girls who ran the sale saw me looking at it. "That's more like five bucks, actually," she said. She'd been talking with her roommate and another young woman who'd stopped by and I hadn't paid much attention to them; now I saw that two of them were fat—they wore their jeans slung low and baggy in characteristic chubby-dyke style; they wore guys' sports shirts. The girl who'd spoken to me was one of the heavy ones.

"It works fine," she said. "You can test it if you want." It had been sitting on a table and I picked it up and set it down just inside the garage. It had a big round dial that went up to 300. I stood on it and watched the needle go up to around 230. I knew the scale was right. I knew also that I ought to buy it. I turned back to the girl.

"It works, huh?" she said.

"It sure does," I said. It was a perfectly good scale. I didn't want to jump to any conclusions about why the women were selling it. But if I were to buy a scale at all, I figured, it might as well be this one. I liked that it was a lesbian scale and that it wouldn't make patriarchal judgments about my weight.

I carried the scale four blocks home, in a plastic grocery bag that almost wasn't strong enough to hold it. The handles cut into my hands and I had to keep stopping and setting it down. The awkwardness didn't matter. It was something I could endure a little longer. Nothing was forever and everything could be measured. It was a matter of 230 pounds on a scale, pounds lined up in a semicircle by fives and tens, little lines like minutes leading up to a present that made sense.

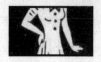

watch

Weight Watchers meetings are held in a beige-walled, windowless basement office space in a modern suburban building that is on my way home from work. The room reminds me, to be honest, of crappy jobs I've had—telemarketing and market research and customer service jobs in rooms like this; jobs with evening hours and shitty, abrasive training sessions run by people with personality disorders. I was afraid my very first Weight Watchers meeting was going to sort of be like that, too.

I've become used to the feeling of stepping on the scale I've bought. It had been so long since I'd stood on one on a regular basis, and it was awkward at first, the way I imagine the Amish would feel on an escalator. But after mastering that step the next thing to do was start Weight Watchers, which I'd chosen sort of arbitrarily. I think I decided on Weight Watchers because I'd been sort of charmed by the Duchess of York in the commercials. In one, she's shown in some kind of mock press conference telling reporters about how much freedom the Weight Watchers plan has, and how you don't have to cut anything out. "So you may *hahve* that banana," she'd said. I loved the sound of her accent when she said *banana*. "You may *hahve* that croissant." She'd had such a rough time in the tabloids, and that whole business with that Texas millionaire, sucking her toes must have been so humiliating when it was in all the papers, so it was really very heartening to see her granting royal permission to eat various food items, very empowering.

I'd found a folding chair near the edge of the room, and after the meeting I was told to stay afterwards with the other newbies to learn how the *1-2-3 POINTS!* system worked. I already knew, having already read all the little fucking booklets. I'd read them carefully throughout the whole meeting, shutting out most of the voices—the testimonials, the applause, the questions—and I'd taken in as much information as I could about points and the relationship of fiber grams to fat and absorbed it into my secret reserve of good intentions, and I didn't want anyone to mess with that. I think I have sort of an odd aversion, almost like a chemical sensitivity, when it comes to other people's enthusiasm.

The orientation was better than I'd thought. Margaret, the leader, explained the way the slide rule worked: you'd use it to calculate calories, fat, and fiber for a point value. "Look," she said, "an apple is one point. You get around twenty-seven points a day. A Burger King Whopper is thirty points." I liked this. It seemed very different from counting calories or following a menu. Calories were messy, visceral data but points felt like something else, like philosophy. It felt shadowless and good.

Plus a girl around my age, a longtime member who'd stayed after to help with the orientation talk, had stood up and very loopily explained how you *so* did not have to buy all the books for the program; how, seriously, you really did need to eat *some* fat, because once she'd tried really, really hard to do fat free *everything* and her hair started to fall out.

"And instead of drinking two or three beers?" she said. "You can get a vodka and cranberry and it's really low in points, *and* you can count the cranberry juice as a daily fruit. Seriously! You *can*." If this had been another low-expectation job instead of a Weight Watchers meeting I would have offered her a Merit Ultra Light during break and tried to be her friend. But instead I grinned at her and picked up all my pamphlets and went home to do my work.

You have to write everything down: your food and your points. At breakfast my cereal and milk and fruit, together, are two points. If I'm good I go around the rest of my day feeling just a little hopped up because the meter is on and ticking and keeping me on duty.

I'm pretty sure the system of consuming no more than twenty-four to twenty-nine points a day is just a simplifying gimmick, but I think I know why I like it so much better than counting calories: the nature of the numbers is different. Calories can measure in the hundreds and are rationed in the thousands and if you think in terms of dollar amounts, the numbers are an awful lot like credit card debt. You start with a limit of eighteen hundred and then max out all too fast. I'm only willing to experience that kind of anxiety in exchange for actual stuff that can be bought at Target. Points, on the other hand, feel more objective: they just *happen*, like the hours in the day.

September 6 I am 229.4 pounds. September 13 I am 227.4. September 20 I'm 227. September 27 I am 226.5. October 4 I'm 225.2. October 11 I don't know because I missed a meeting. October 18 I'm 222.3 October 25 I'm 222. November 1 I get an *I lost 5 pounds!* bookmark even though the loss did not technically occur on November 1. I'm 222.1. November 8 I'm 220.1.

But sometimes I still get lost inside a day and will try to stop time by not eating, or else I'll lose pockets of time here and there, intervals in which I might have eaten something—*what?*—or else I'll eat and hope the minutes extend long enough to get me somewhere else altogether.

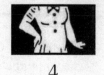

how many cups are in a typical order of pad thai, according to angelkara33 on the weightwatchers.com bulletin boards

Hi I usually try to have a salad w/ ff or lo-cal dressing first then I take a look at the plate when it arrives. It's really not that hard to visualize how much 1 cup would be, imagine your plate at home and how much it would have on it. I think in the back of the WW book it gives some tips on how to estimate portions. I am not tempted anymore to eat much more than 1 or 1½ cup portions anymore and I am finding it easier now to ask how food is prepared and request less oil, etc. One thing you can do to reduce the guilt/points is to avoid deep-fried food! (I love lomein from my Chinese restaurant and ask them to make it with half the usual oil, it still tastes great). If the restaurant doesn't have salad (Thai is a good example) try having some clear or veg. soup before you start on the entree. That way when you start the main course you shouldn't feel so starved and that 1 or 2 pts on soup/salad is usually a lot less than eating double or triple portions. And the bonus is you can take the rest home and eat 1–2 more meals from leftovers.:) I've lost 25 pds. on WW since Sept, and have eaten out many times. Also when in doubt stay on the low side of your pts for the rest of the day, and try not to use banked pts for a few more days, that way if you did go over (it can be hard to estimate restaurant food), you should still be okay. I have found I lose more when I'm conservative on estimating pts. Good luck!

Oh, for fuck's sake. I'd posted a simple question. I hate the Internet.

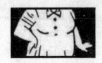

predestination

I didn't really have a gruesome Fat Childhood; nothing that I can offer as an explanation. When I was in first grade all you had to do was look at me funny and I'd cry. I'd bawl and wail and my little sandals would fall off and I'd accidentally drop my paper-plate flower art project in a puddle or something. Not always necessarily in that order; but either way, any way, the world would frequently and without warning spin itself into a hot glaring maelstrom and nothing could console me, because I was on my own personal crap carousel and I couldn't get it to stop. Other kids noticed. Teachers and lunchroom ladies noticed. They kept the carousel going, and I was a pretty miserable little shit.

My mom talked to my teacher and somehow they decided it was because I wasn't used to being at school all day and I'd get hungry and cranky and sensitive. I was told all this; it *did* sort of help to know that I was the wimpiest child who ever lived. The solution was to give me a snack in the middle of the afternoon, so at an appointed time I'd get rounded up with two older kids to go to the nurse's office and have a snack. There was a diabetic girl, some other kid whose problem I didn't know, and me. One of them got graham crackers; the other, a piece of fruit.

My snacks were very special. They were these chewy chocolate sticks, very modular looking, individually wrapped, and they had a vague nutritional legitimacy about them. I understand they used to be called Space Food Sticks in the '60s, and people are now very nostalgic about them, but I think when I had them in the '70s they were called, simply, Food Sticks. They were frankly utilitarian and yet so chocolately, and I truly enjoyed the sense of importance with which I ate them.

And they must have dropped the "Space" from the name by the time the Food Sticks came into my life, because I can pretty clearly recall what the box looked like, the way it had a little Pillsbury logo, and how it was kept in a cabinet of the nurse's office. I know I would have remembered the "Space" part had it been there. It would have been a good word to go with how strange it felt to leave a classroom and go into a quiet room and wait shyly until they fed me something. Then I had to go back up the stairs by myself.

After school on Tuesdays, starting in second grade, I'd go with my friend Colette Molloy and her mother to church, to a Christian youth group. Somehow I'd talked my agnostic parents into letting me go there, and I went almost every week for two school years. It was called Pioneer Girls, and it appeared to be run by a group of parents.

Mrs. Molloy usually brought cookies—economy packages of sandwich cookies or waffle crèmes. The chocolate ones were a little like the Figurines diet bars my mom would buy but wouldn't let me eat, even though they were sometimes the only remotely cookie-ish thing in the house. In this way I came to count on Pioneer Girls. We'd eat the cookies and have Bible study groups and do craft projects—Noah's Arks out of Popsicle sticks, maybe—and then gather together at the end to sing songs.

I liked Pioneer Girls at first, but by the time I was in fourth grade, I could get away with sneaking off and wandering around the church, looking in the nursery rooms, the supply closets, the kitchen. I was bored. And it wasn't my church.

In the refrigerator, which always had a rancid cabbage smell, I found a can of Reddi-wip. For weeks I kept going back for handfuls of whipped cream. A couple times I even took the can to a little hallway off the kitchen where I could eat it without getting caught.

At Pioneer Girls we learned that God decided everything we would ever do in our lifetimes. Mrs. Reece had explained it with a particular emphasis on the *evers*. "*Every*thing *every*one in the whole entire world *ever* did throughout all time," she said, "or will *ever* do in the history of the world, was all thought up by God. He decided all of it before the world was ever even created." When she said this I could see Mrs. Molloy nodding across the room. I knew I was supposed to believe Mrs. Reece but I didn't.

I didn't believe, but week after week I went to the re-frigerator, thinking that whatever I found or did not find would have a meaning. Once or twice it occurred to me that maybe I should just *not* eat the stuff, but I was waiting for a sign. I was waiting to look in the fridge and find that the Reddi-wip was gone.

But what happened is that I finished off the whole can, and then I put it back where I'd found it. And after an-other week, I went back to make sure it was still empty, and then I threw it out.

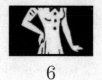

6

it's your body it's your world

From the looks of the television commercials, the Women's Workout World gym is a reasonably empowering kind of place, I guess. It shows women in taut sports tanks pushing and pulling things on chrome machines. One woman working the chest press has her chin lifted and her eyes staring a thousand miles into the distance, like a Soviet heroine. "It's your body," sings the throaty, almost diva-esque jingle singer. "It's your world."

It's a world with considerably less ass showing than in the trashy Bally's commercials and you have to appreciate that. It's a world where women step in unison with fist-clenching, bicep-flexing arm movements. And it looks almost cool, like Bitch Army basic training. I figure if I'm going to join a gym, it might as well be this one.

The Women's Workout World gym that I attend used to be a Treasure Island supermarket. You can tell by the big open space inside, by the one wall of windows that run across the front of the place where the checkout counters must have been. There are abdominal benches there now.

The décor is very '80s: the walls are teal and purple, with teal and purple neon tubes running above all the mirrors. I like this, as it looks exactly like the sort of health club I figured I'd attend one day, back when I was thinking of these things in 1983 and imagining myself in various outfits against the appropriate settings, trying to conjure up my grown-up self like some kind of Aspirational Barbie who'd go from a navy blue skirted suit and a silvery glass office backdrop to a smartly striped leotard, a pair of leg warmers, and a place, yes, *just like* Women's Workout World.

Going there takes some getting used to. I go through a brief StairMaster phase for about a week and half, until a couple of girls I talk to at my friend Leigh's Halloween party tell me that doing the StairMaster "doesn't work," though they don't explain how. "It just . . . *doesn't*," one of them says.

"Yeah, it's really bad," her friend says. They are both dressed as cheerleaders. Ironic cheerleaders, but still, they look like they know their gym stuff. I'd come dressed as Little Debbie and clearly I don't.

The StairMaster sucks but I figure other things ought to work. I spend a lot of time on the treadmill, and learn to stay away from Treadmill Three because the handrail gives off one hell of a static electricity shock. I try taking the classes. I like Cardio Kickboxing, because it makes me feel like Pussy Galore, and I am trying to like Step Aerobics.

Eventually I go there at least twice a week, and I change into a long T-shirt and a pair of sweatpants and put my hair in a bandanna, and I go out on the aerobics floor and stand there and wait for the Step I class to begin. There are mirrors along three of the walls; some of the women use them to stretch, or to check their form while they use the free weights. I'm not really sure what I should be doing in the mirrors while waiting like this. I get caught up in all the deliberate motion that I can see reflected behind me—the machines and the girls on them, and the women who are just coming in with their street clothes still on. I follow their coats; I watch a few of them and try to figure out whether they're students at Loyola or Eastern, or if they're working professionals; if they work downtown; if they're my age. Sometimes the women look something like what I thought I would have grown up to be, and when I catch myself standing there I consider whether there's any resemblance or whether I'm just someone else now.

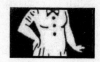

princess shit

Today on my desk at work there is a little card I have to fill out indicating whether I want the chicken, steak, or fish entree at the company Christmas party and also whether I'll be bringing a guest. This year the answers are *chicken* and *no*, though in the past I've had steak.

Also on my desk are a stack of manuscripts that I read in between surfing the Internet. Call me a slacker, but I used to post so often on this one *Dawson's Creek* bulletin board that when the women who ran it decided to start a site that's now called Television Without Pity, they invited me to join the staff. Now, occasionally, I get paid to write a funny review of a really crappy television drama, and, of course, they were my excuse to go to Las Vegas.

But I still have to keep my day job, which is at a small publishing company. I read unsolicited children's book manuscript submissions. We get a lot of them because it is apparently the dream of at least every third person in America to publish a children's book. My job, much to my perpetual relief, does not require a childlike sense of wonder. I figured that out from Alice and Karen, the other two editors, who have been with the company more than twenty years.

Alice calls from her office. "I have learned the true meaning of Christmas *at last*." She's going through the manuscripts, too.

"Really?" I yell back. "What did the Brave Little Christmas Tree That Nobody Wanted teach you *this* time?"

You really shouldn't get us started.

This week I have come across at least three princess manuscripts so far. This is pretty typical: people like to write princess stories, I guess. Today's is about a princess who won't brush her teeth, but I've also read ones about princesses whose mean fathers won't let them study engineering; princesses who don't even know they're princesses; and princesses who get along *just fine* with their stepmothers, *thank you very much*.

They are not usually fairy tales. In fact, they're most often perfectly ordinary stories that just happen to take place in a castle with a few royal something-or-others thrown in for fun—a royal minivan, for instance. People think that's sort of funny. The feeling I always get when I read these, is that the writers have no idea how to tell a story about a real girl, so they make her a princess and they give her a predicament.

* * *

On my way home from work I stop at my Weight Watchers meeting. We have gotten a late November snow—wet and showy in the morning, mixed with sleet in the evening. Walking through the parking lot I am chilly and wet and tired; I wish I had a big warm loaf of bread the size of a Honda Civic, so that I could chew my way inside and fall asleep in it.

The line is longer than usual because Weight Watching citizens are panicking about the coming Thanksgiving holiday. Also, the sign-in process for Weight Watchers is painfully elaborate. They have booklets and folders and file cards; there are stickers and stamps and check marks and secret handshakes, practically. I am pretty sure the receptionist is dead inside in order to be able to do this. Or this might be her occupational therapy.

When I finally get to the scale to weigh in, it shows that I haven't lost at all. I am up slightly: 220.3. I think I must be wearing too many heavy layers of clothes to get a decent reading—too many heavy, damp, itchy layers of clothing that I never much liked in the first place. I don't stay for the stupid meeting, and I have to shuffle the last few steps back to my car because things are starting to freeze.

I try not to feel sorry for myself as I drive home. I decide I will not feel worthless. I will not act like I'm the Cracked Ceramic Unicorn Nobody Wanted—though seriously, someone has written that story and sent it to the place where I work.

I am fine. I am not a princess. I mean, *fuck* that princess shit, I am thinking. I am getting practically every red light between Touhy and Devon and my car's transmission does not like this one bit, and fuck that princess shit.

Single is a princess word. *What a pretty face you have* is a princess phrase. Being fat is bad enough without it being a stupid princess predicament where I'm supposed to bust out of my pumpkin shell one day and break my own stupid spell and be pretty and happy ever after—and really, fuck that, I think, all the way home.

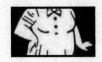

your momma

I don't know how much my mother weighs now, or how much she usually weighed while I was growing up, or what was the most that she ever weighed. I look at pictures and at the tags on her clothes (size 26 maybe?) and I will stand next to her, but I can't come up with more than a *something somewhere*; maybe a three-hundred-something God knows when; maybe more, maybe not now. She's almost always been fat.

I was maybe around eight years old when I needed her to help me with some homework—some kind of demented assignment like "Describe Someone," which required me to use adjectives. "My mom looks like . . ." I wrote. "Brown curly hair, glasses." I read it out loud to her as I formed the words on paper. I put down *brown eyes*. "Right?" I asked. I remember being somehow too shy to determine things like that. I could look at eyes but I needed someone to verify the color—to me, a person's eyes were too intimate and strange to have fixed properties like that.

"Right," my mom said. I wrote it down. I needed more. I started another sentence with "She is . . ."

I read it back to her and looked up. "Plump?" I tried.

"Oh, God," my mom said. "Just write down *fat*." I wanted to laugh because she was laughing, sort of. At that age a lot of my life was divided into places where my mom would let me go and places where she wouldn't. I didn't know where this was.

"Am I supposed to say that?" I asked.

"Tell them your mother is fat." She sounded almost insistent.

Once when I was a little younger, we'd been at Rehm Park Pool, and she'd been floating on her back near me in the shallow section. I was in waist-deep: the waterline hit right where my hands felt most useful, and I kept running my hands back and forth, smoothing the little currents; the surface was like a big table and my mom was right there on it. I waded over and looked down. I knew how her tummy felt if I rubbed it; I was fascinated by the way wet swimsuit fabric felt—one of those goofy tactile kid fetishes—and my mom had plenty of it that I could touch. It was funny to have her lying down this way in the same place I was standing, and I slipped my hands under her. I thought this was brilliant. I balanced my mom's body against my palms and felt like I'd changed the laws of everything.

"Look!" I yelled out, to no one in particular. "I'm lifting my mom and she's big and fat!"

When she dunked me I had still been shouting. When I went under it felt like all the sound had been sucked back into my head through my ears.

When I came back up she'd said, "Do you know why I did that?"

That time I knew why. But I didn't know why she was doing what she was doing now, with my homework paper.

I wrote: "She is plump (Fat)."

I didn't really know what parentheses were but I had an idea about how to use them: you'd write a lazy forward C and then a backward one; you did it for the things you needed to both say and not say.

#

the perfect fat girl

She can't quite be you but she can never be too fat or sad to haunt your story. She can be a ghost. (Though at her size, weightlessness doesn't count.) She can be lost, or else she can be looking for the body she lost. Maybe the body has amnesia and she's waiting to bring it back to her senses. Whose senses? It's easy to forget. All she remembers is waking up fat.

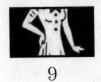

9

success story

My therapist is named Elizabeth, and I like her shoes, especially the wedge-heel Mary Janes she wears sometimes with tights. We meet once a week in an office that she borrows from another therapist: a room with a decent second-hand couch and lots of plants and an old wooden file cabinet that I plan to steal one day. There are little pieces of folk art and some kind of colorful abstract glass art object that I find myself wanting to put in my mouth, and while it's a bizarre thought, it's probably not one that's completely out of place in a therapist's office either. I like to think that out of all of Elizabeth's clients, I'm the most special and she likes me best of all. She would never say that of course, but *I bet*.

I'm relieved Elizabeth is no longer pregnant. When I first started sessions with her back in the spring, a few months before the Vegas trip, she was just beginning her third trimester, and as the weeks went by I began to get sort of alarmed at the sight of her in an office task chair. She'd shift her weight under her big pumpkin belly and urge me to talk about my body issues and here I wasn't even the one who was about to have *a person come out of her headfirst*. I can concentrate a little better now that she's had the baby.

Currently, we're working on why I think I'm kind of worthless. For now, Elizabeth and I are putting aside the matter of the answers themselves in order to sort out the accompanying disclaimers and fine print. For instance I suppose I think I'm kind of worthless *because I'm fat*, but you have to take into consideration things like subhead 2: *It could be worse*; and 2.1: *It's not like people point at me on the street or anything*; and 2.2(c.): *For Christ's sake, I don't have an eating disorder*; and also 3.2(a.): *I guess I avoid relationships and stuff*; and 3.2(b): *Or they avoid me*; as well as 4: *I don't even read those magazines*; 4.3: *And everyone says Renee Zellweger looks hotter in that one movie*; and, not least of all, 5: *Seriously, I know I'm not completely worthless*; and 5.1: *Because, after all, I am here*. Right, Elizabeth?

Sometimes she buys that. But I can only suck up to her so much, shoe compliments notwithstanding. "You've come so far," she says. "And what else can you do to feel better?" she asks.

That's a difficult question to answer. I look at the crooked slat near the top of the blinds in the window closest to me here in the borrowed office, and then at the paint blister near the ceiling. In the past seven months my eyes have picked out all kinds of little difficult-question places around the room. When I go to them, my mind checks all the fuses. I have been losing weight and, if it is a means to an end, I don't know quite where that end *goes*.

I should tell Elizabeth that I've lost almost ten pounds and that I've gone to the gym four times this past week, but I don't want to say those are the things that will make me feel better. Because of course they're not. *Right, Elizabeth?*

Weight Watchers Magazine has surprisingly classy recipes and the cover often features Sarah, Duchess of York, wearing dress shirts tailored to show off her waist. Every dozen pages or so there's a Success Story showing a large picture of the successful person in a kicky new outfit and a smaller inset photo of the person when he or she was fatter. Jennifer Biester, 27, is a real estate agent who ate too much fast food on the go; now she carries healthy low-*POINTS* snacks with her at all times. Evelyn DeRosta, 36, has taken up daily walking and has found delicious alternatives to the rich foods she used to cook for her family.

At first, I have trouble imagining what the set-up or initial premise of my Success Story would be, other than I just eat too fucking much. But then, I know that the Weight Watchers euphemism for that problem is *portion control* and that my tendency to go through a whole take-out order of Pad Kee Mao noodles could be simply alluded to in the phrase *busy city single-gal lifestyle*, though that might in turn be a little too closely associated with tipped-back Cosmopolitans and blow jobs in cabs. But then again, a Success Story life probably means lots of things are open to interpretation.

* * *

"Maybe I should write about this stuff," I am telling Elizabeth. I have been searching my mind trying to think of What Else I Can Do to Feel Better, and this is all I can come up with. I don't have a story; I just want what happens to be a story.

"That's good," she says. "Keep a journal, you mean?"

Well, no. When I try to keep a private written journal it's kind of a disaster, what with my psychotic handwriting and the sometimes unfortunate free-form Natalie Goldberg habits I cultivated in college, the ones that cause me to write things like *do I what but follow inevitably thus thought blur the forest*. Instead, I tell her, I thought I'd put it all on a website or something.

Elizabeth nods. "So other people can read about it?"

"I guess," I say. But I hadn't really thought about other people. I just want my stuff on a computer screen and therefore in the same place as everything else I know or want to know or am about to know. I want it to be behind the glass.

Elizabeth thinks this is a good idea. It would be even better if I knew how to build a website.

I have been meaning to learn how to put up one of these things pretty much the same way I have been meaning to be not so fat. So I have to teach myself a few things. I go by trial and error and also by something called "Netscape Composer," an application that makes horrible things happen sometimes.

Sometimes making and putting up the pages feels like

painting backward on a window. I don't know how to make colors work: somehow, the colors are numbers. I don't understand why a page looks perfectly fine on my desktop but then shows up as lines and lines of garble online. Words and boxes will suddenly fall apart or disintegrate into bits of code—*&sp;< b*—that look like cartoon profanity. Images, especially, are a pain: they have a habit of turning into plain gray boxes when I upload the page; they somehow go bad like cheap lightbulbs.

I learn slowly. I manage to put up a page, one where I'd written about my day, and my day was about going to the gym. Or else it was about how I did twenty-five minutes on the treadmill at the gym at a speed of 3.5 and an incline level of 4; or it was about watching one of the older women at the gym, a woman from Europe, wearing not quite the right shoes and pedaling slowly on one of the stationary bicycles, nodding to herself a little; I didn't really know why she was riding the way she was, or, really, what she was trying to accomplish and whether the effort lived in her legs or her mind or some other part, but then, maybe it was enough that she was there; perhaps being there could be worth something to her or to me, even if I didn't know what else to do besides mention some of it in passing—the woman, the shoes, the gym where I went that day.

I figure out how to put up another page and link back to the first one and I write another day's worth of stuff there, too. I do this a few more times until there's something where I can click from one page to the next and make all the days work.

For a while it's enough that all the days link to each other. Nobody needs to read the pages; I just like knowing that they work.

i know cathy

It's Christmas and we're opening presents. The extended family—uncles, aunts, cousins—have come over to my mom and dad's place for dessert and for the gift exchange. I'm not terribly close with the relatives who have driven down from St. Paul; on Christmas, the Minnesota Michaelsons wear nice Fair Isle sweaters with lots of red in them, and they always have celebrated Christmas the way I used to want my parents to do it, with a real tree and a fireplace. I guess a little bit of me still wants to play along with this Perfect Christmas notion because I always find myself picking out gifts for each one of them: my cousin, her husband, their three children. And every year I forget that they, the Minnesota Michaelsons, have always given me only *one* thing—"from all of us," my cousin Trish will say. This year it's in a little jewelry box.

I open it and inside, wrapped in tissue paper, is a *Cathy*

pin. A big, pewter rectangular pin the size of, well, of a Sunday paper comic strip panel, because clearly the intended charm of this novelty jewelry creation is that it's a *Cathy* comic strip panel reimagined in pewter for the sake of posterity and "laughs."

My cousin looks over from across the room and sees that I have opened the box. "Did you see it?" she calls. "It's Cathy." I'm looking under the tissue paper to see if there's anything else, but indeed there is only one thing, *and it's Cathy.*

Cartoon Cathy is engraved in her trademark doodle-y lines on the shiny pewter surface: she is googly-eyed, and her hair looks a little frazzled, and she's wearing a career woman blazer, and she's saying, "AAAACK!!!" I'm not sure why. I understand that Cathy has disgorged a speech balloon full of AAAACK on more than one occasion in the twenty-something-year history of her comic strip. But she's not depicted in a department store dressing room here, and she's not sitting in front of a pie; she's just sitting there at her desk. I'm guessing that this is more of an existential AAAACK.

"It just reminds me of you," my cousin Trish says. "Ha! You know?" I think she can tell that I'm not thrilled. I'm trying to hide it. "Not that you're necessarily this big *Cathy* fan or anything," she says. "But it's just . . . it seems like something *you'd* say, or just, you know, how you can be sometimes, just—*funny.*"

I know it's supposed to be a compliment.

I wish I could better explain what my problem is with *Cathy.* Really, on any given day on the funny pages *Cathy* isn't so bad; Cathy usually manages to flail her way toward one relevant cultural truth or another. You can't put your finger on any one thing that is ideologically wrong with a *Cathy* cartoon and Cathy would not be the worst person in the world to sit next to on a Greyhound bus. When it comes down to it, the only thing that's wrong with Cathy is that *she won't go away*. I have childhood memories of reading *Cathy*, of her complaining about the Scarsdale Diet and *aaaack*ing while trying on blouses with huge shoulder pads. My mom had a clipped *Cathy* strip on the bulletin board in the kitchen. In it Cathy was talking to her friend Andrea about carbohydrates and I think the joke had something to do with the absurdity of talking about carbohydrates. To grow up reading *Cathy* is to understand on some subliminal level that *Cathy* is about perpetual wretchedness and senseless, pigheaded stupidity. I mean, Jesus Christ, just because the fashion industry will always make unflattering swimsuits *does not mean you have to try every last one of them on*, but Cathy does, and I hate her for that. That thing she's struggling to pull up around her ass isn't a thong; it's an *infinite loop*. It's never going to fit. I get it, I *understand*. I've understood ever since I was at least fourteen. And I'd managed to shut out most of the pathos (Cathos?) until now.

I look down at the pin. "Thanks," I say. "I mean . . . yeah. I know *Cathy*." I am almost thirty and it occurs to me that I'm now old enough to be someone Cathy supposedly represents; somehow I've stumbled into her scary forever world.

"I hope you like it," says my cousin, a little nervously.

*   *   *

Most of our Christmas dessert consists of stuff ordered from the Swiss Colony catalog: petits fours, marzipan, chocolate-covered toffee and Dobosh torte. My grand-mother likes to order these things. Somehow she doesn't have the family weight problem, despite a raging sweet tooth that she's nurtured for so many years she can point out where all the Fannie May candy shops are on a Chicago map. She hasn't been downtown in a decade but sometimes I will call out an intersection: "Quincy and Wells, Grandma. Where's the closest Fannie May?" and she'll get it right. She likes Fannie May best, See's is "shitty," and Swiss Colony makes some decent pastries. I have to agree.

When I was a kid I loved the Swiss Colony catalogs. I would flip through the pages and pretend that I was a lit-tle match girl taken in by rich benefactors—not exactly a Daddy Warbucks kind of arrangement, because I always thought that was creepy, but maybe a couple of shut-in ec-centric old ladies who depended on catalogs to satisfy their lavish whims, and that's how, at Christmas, I would get to invite all my orphan friends to a two-day feast made up en-tirely of Swiss Colony food. Breakfast with honey ham and pancakes; premium steaks for lunch; sausage appetizers; smoked turkey dinner; Jelly Roll Yule Log cake for dessert—*all* the shit. You could throw a fruit basket in there somewhere so it would be nutritionally balanced. But it would be amazing. I'd imagine how it would all look to one of the guest orphans I'd invited, what with five-pound chocolate sculptures and ten kinds of spreadable cheese. It would be *so* extravagant that the orphans would nearly faint at the sight of the spread. But then they'd learn to enjoy the food carefully, without getting too pathetic and desperate and gross.

It pretty much goes without saying I have to call on my sense of Orphan Self-Control tonight.

I have lost more than fifteen pounds now, and today, on Christmas, some people are starting to notice—the people who tend to notice these things, at least; mostly the older women. One of my grandmother's cousins says, "You're getting so *skinny!*" I'm a little bothered by hyperbole like that. If people tell me I'm "skinny" when I'm still over 200 pounds, I wonder if they mean they don't have a *word* for what I am; that I was just so fat before that nuances escape them and thus they must invoke the binary opposite of how I used to look.

I shouldn't think about this kind of thing too much, but I do.

For now I still want to appear to be proceeding quietly and gracefully—just *reducing*, as the older relatives say, which is an appealing word to me, since something that is reduced tends not to only be smaller but simpler as well. Every now and then I get up from the living room—even, once, the dinner table—just to walk around the house because, well, I don't know: maybe I'm just getting so thin that I am compelled to float around or something. Whatever force used to keep me sitting in the recliner isn't as strong; it could be that I'm becoming reduced enough to experience subtler bodily impulses like *turn just enough to make your stomach muscles taut* and *put your shoulders back and stretch*, and of course I have to see how something like that looks, and that's why I'll be by the hall mirror sometimes—no other reason, really.

things i tell the mostly imaginary readers of my website

That the low-point crustless pumpkin pie substitute that gets recommended at Weight Watchers meetings tastes like aspartame and ass; that a two-ounce, three-point serving of turkey is so fucking small that it can be accidentally inhaled; how I'm disproportionately annoyed with abbreviations like "ff" for "fat-free," and how losing weight has gotten harder after the first round of compliments because going on feels vaguely improper, like staying at a party too long.

That today's poor lunchtime choice of a Thai noodle entrée was due to the morning's various unforeseen and completely annoying events such as a broken bra underwire and a problem with the hot water heater in my apartment building; how my favorite part of *Charlie and the Chocolate Factory* was when Violet Beauregarde chews that gum that provides the sensation of eating a full meal, and how I wished it really existed because gum doesn't make you fat. I want to change my body and I want to be shallow and I want to be a fairy princess and I tell everyone this, or at the very least I experience *the sensation* of telling everyone.

I get to tell everyone that I've lost fifteen pounds. Just, you know, in passing.

My friend Michael from college (and my housemate from that one hyper summer) is reading my site—all six pages of it—from North Carolina after one night on the phone I'd told him I was writing again. I think a couple of people from the Television Without Pity staff have seen the site. My friend Richard knows my site exists but he never reads stuff on the computer. However, he did say that now that I've lost weight he can totally see my boobs now. "Maybe you could be one of those webcam girls!" he says over drinks at Little Nut Hut, and I will take that as some kind of encouragement.

In one of our sessions Elizabeth says, "Am I going to get to see it?"

"Um, good question," I say. I mean, I wonder what she thinks is on my site. The other day I wrote about how I spent my entire step class pretending I was on an episode of *Pop Stars*: I did all the moves imagining that I was nineteen years old and had a pierced navel and I was auditioning for the break of a lifetime. Would the things that I wrote affect our subsequent appointments? Would Elizabeth say stuff like, *Tell me more about wanting to be in a group like Destiny's Child; where do you think that feeling comes from?*

"But, you know, don't feel that you need to show it to me," she adds. "Unless you somehow think it's necessary for me to understand what's going on with you."

"Well, I think so far I've been doing a pretty good job of just *telling* you, right?" Sometimes it seems like that's all that happens in our sessions: I'll sit down on the lumpy couch and talk and meaningfully explicate and answer my own questions and provide helpful metaphors for a good twenty minutes before I let her take a crack at my problems. And, in fact, today I find myself explaining to Elizabeth that I think I'm doing this whole crazy site in the first place in order to grant myself a feeling of self-possession because I've concluded that my deep reluctance to tell people I'm trying to get into shape has less to do with wanting to keep it secret than it does with how I don't want to give myself over to everyone else's opinions on *how big my ass should be* and hence my productive activity in the form of this online journal. Which I'll let Elizabeth read, because, well, why not?

"But I'm *not* going to use it as way to somehow communicate with you outside of this office," I point out.

"I think that's fine," says Elizabeth.

"Because that probably wouldn't be healthy," I tell her. "I mean, it would be pretty fucked-up if I did that."

Since everyone who reads my site knows me, it seems a little goofy and redundant to keep calling my site *Wendy's*

Most Fabulous Page, which I'd typed at the top of the index page to let all five people know they'd come to the right place and also so I could play with HTML and see how big "*<font size=7>*" made the letters. (Pretty fucking big.) But now my site needs some other kind of name, I guess. A title, even, although I don't want to make any assumptions as to what kind of story I'm living.

I suppose the name should have something to do with weight loss, since mostly I'm writing about that and not my job or my observations about '80s music videos, which in my real life I tend to discuss a hell of a lot more often than I do my own weight. But this site is just about this one part of me, or the whole of me that I hardly ever want to mention.

No way am I going to call it something like *My Weight Loss Journey*, for fuck's sake. Or *Losin' It*. Or *Weigh to Go!* Or *Soon to Be Slender*, or *Road to Fitness*, or anything that contains the words *goal, challenge, quest, thin, before & after*, the use of the phrase construction *from _____ to _____*; the use of "2" as a variation on "to" in the aforementioned example or really in any context that is not a hip-hop song title; puns on *weight, lose, skinny, fat*, and most especially for the love of all that is holy, *phat*.

I think about calling the site *My Body Journal* but it sounds too somber, or like lame erotica. *Funky Flesh* has bad B.O. connotations. For about two hours I love *Punk Rock Will Never DieT* until I finally admit to myself that I am not very punk rock and indeed, I *am* on a diet.

Every title I can think of has words that I don't use unless absolutely necessary: slim, scale, weigh, et cetera.

When I talk about my weight at all it's simply to mention the pounds I've lost. I think that's all I care about, and as it's the pure science part—the measurements, the units, the evidence of change, it's the only part I know for sure isn't completely bullshit. Plus I like that *pound* is not just a noun, though I have no idea how to wield it as a verb for my own purposes. I don't know who or what I'd *pound* and with what, and why. But I like that the potential to do so is there in the word somehow, like an energy principle in physics. So that's what I call my site: *Pound*.

"What about your family?" Elizabeth asks me. By that she means my mother. "Do they know?"

"About the site? No," I say. Elizabeth doesn't ask me to explain why, though I usually do. "No," I say again, and leave it at that.

skin

I spend one of my days off after Christmas at my parents' house, where we are trying to organize a ton of old family pictures. The photographs are completely out of order and most of them belong to my grandmother, who has been meaning to get them in order for at least as long as she has been collecting unused photo albums, photo boxes with file tabs, drawers with special clear plastic photo sleeves you can flip through like a card catalog, and a brass contraption that looks kind of like a big Rolodex file, only for your photos. Photograph storage contraptions are, to my grandmother, pretty much what diet books, workout tapes, and Weight Watchers recipe cards are to my mother, and now all of their well-intentioned crap is together in one ranch house basement. Now that my grandmother lives with my parents, we've come to realize that no matter what the Next Big Thing in Photo Organization is, it's really not going to help the situation.

So we've taken this day to go through some of the boxes and we've sat Grandma down at the dining room table so that we can hold up pictures and ask her about them. There are snapshots from my dad's childhood mixed in with photos of my grandma's trip to Europe in 1985. There are cousins and obscure relatives that only my grandmother knows, and also a truly alarming number of pictures of people nobody knows anymore. We are mostly just trying to find ourselves in them.

We have been at this for about an hour now. We have two piles: Known and Unknown, and my dad is fishing through Known for duplicates.

In the handful of pictures I've pulled out of one of the boxes, there is a picture of a baby, and behind the baby there is a woman on the couch whose head is mostly out of the frame. It could be a picture of me but it's hard to tell because of the way the baby's head is turned.

"Mom, is this me? This baby?" I ask, handing it to her. She says it isn't and hands it back. I look at it some more. The date stamp on the edge of the photo says 1971. I look at the woman in the background. It could be anyone but it could also be her.

"Are you sure?" I ask. I walk back over and show it to her. "Isn't this you on the couch?" My mom stares at it. "You know . . . it could be," she said. "The date would be right, and I know I was pretty skinny after I had you . . ." We decide it must be us.

After that, I start looking through the photos for glimpses of my mom—her back, in a sleeveless dress at an anniversary party; her arm resting on the dinner table at

our house on Christmas. Or maybe just her face somewhere and I try to figure out the body from the face.

In a few pictures it's all I can do to figure out the body
because of the surgeries my mom has had. She has had her
stomach stapled twice. The first time I was in fifth grade;
she'd had her gall bladder out and the doctor talked her
into trying the staples, too. She did it again six months
later. She hadn't lost enough weight the first time, she
thought.

The second time was more successful. That summer
we'd taken a car trip to New Mexico and the photograph I
am holding now shows her posing with my great-aunt at a
scenic overlook. She was wearing khaki shorts and a green
halter top. What I notice the most is the way her skin
crumpled around the tops of her legs and hung beneath her
arms. She was a size 14, and she had the extra skin; she'd
lost nearly 100 pounds and she wouldn't gain it back for a
few more years. She was finishing graduate school and
would soon start working as a therapist, where she'd help
other people with their problems. It seemed fitting, now
that she no longer embodied a problem herself.

In the picture she is grinning so wide she could have
been laughing. Her skin didn't fit her anymore; that's the
thing in the picture I can't stop noticing, so it almost seems
like she could be laughing at that—some joke about the fat
lady who's not there anymore. Or maybe the joke was on
everyone else: everyone who thought my mother would be
something else under her fat—something different, finally—but as it turned out, she was skin.

I put the photo in the Known pile and continue.

a long way, baby

Just to prove I can be spontaneous once in a while I take only three minutes to put on mascara and a clean sweater and then I walk five blocks to the Davis theater. My friends Leigh and Richard are waiting there with cigarettes and guilty looks on their faces. The *Charlie's Angels* movie is sold out.

"Oh shit," says Leigh. "The one time you actually decide to come." They'd gotten their tickets already. Leigh's known me for years and knows I don't tend to do stuff on short notice.

"It's okay," I tell them. It's a warm night, and it's early, and now that I'm out here, I decide I can hang out for a couple of hours and meet them for drinks after the movie. Really, it's fine.

"You'll be, like, our fallen Angel," says Leigh. She and Richard vow they'll miss me the way the whole wide world missed Farrah Fawcett when she left the original show and was replaced.

"*Fuck* Cheryl Ladd," says Richard.

I go across the street and kill some time browsing at the record store until it closes. Then I get a newspaper and go to the bar where we've agreed to meet. Ricochet's is a dark neighborhood bar that has made some effort to offset the slightly dive-ish atmosphere with decorative touches like green banker's lamps, a couple of plants, and a framed Anne Geddes baby poster in the ladies' room that I know is intended to make us gals feel more at home even as it makes me want to smash things. But for the most part Ricochet's is okay.

It's pretty quiet there now, and the end of the bar counter where I am sitting is empty, or it is until a guy with an untucked WISCONSIN T-shirt comes in and sits a few stools down. I turn back to reading but in my peripheral vision I can tell when he moves around. He turns on his stool to look all around the bar and he seems a little restless. He gets up again and goes over to the jukebox. When he sits down again he's closer to me.

"So, I'm going to play some music. Any requests?" he asks.

"Um . . . no," I tell him. I'm being called on to banter and I'm really not up for it right now.

"You sure?"

"Yeah."

"I'm Terry," he says and wants to shake hands. I shake his and tell him my name. "You need a drink, Lindy?" he says, getting my name wrong.

"No, but thanks."

"I'm not going to bug you if I play music, am I?" he asks.

"No."

"Because you seem really busy reading that paper."

"I'm fine," I say. I know I'm being Solitary While Female, a serious offense in bars sometimes, but come on.

He doesn't go away at first. He's stood up but I can tell he is lingering there and looking around some more. He goes down to the end of the bar where the bartender is and talks to him. Then he walks back and grabs his jacket and says, "I'll be right back." I kind of hope not. He walks out the side door of the bar.

I check the time. It's about 9:15 and the movie is supposed to let out around 10:30.

When he comes back in he's got his hands full. He's got a large Slurpee from the 7-Eleven down the street; an empty cup for a small Slurpee; and a pack of cigarettes. He returns to his seat at the bar and he orders a shot of Ketel One. I watch as he pours some red Slurpee from the big cup to the small one, and then he picks up the shot glass and pours the vodka in. He stirs everything with the long plastic spoon and puts a straw in it. And then he drinks it. He's picking up his cigarettes and rapping the box against the bar to pack them. They're Virginia Slims.

"So . . ." he says.

No, really, he lights one. It's a 100. He's smoking it.

"Lindy, right?" he asks.

"Wendy," I correct him.

"I'm still Terry," he says.

"Yes, you are."

While I read the paper he watches the TV over the bar. There's some kind of cable news on and he purposefully wonders out loud: "Where's that happening?" and "Did they say if the Cubs won?" I shrug a lot. I guess I could go somewhere else for a while but Terry seems pretty harmless. He looks to be about my age; his face is nice, though a little heavyset and not quite right for the haircut he's got. I keep hearing him suck spiked Slurpee through his straw. I would like to think that truly crazy people do not give themselves away like this.

He wants to know if I play pool; I don't, not really. Do I want to help him pick out songs on the jukebox? Am I sure I don't want a drink? I achieve a perverse joy in being no fun at all.

"Okay," I say, finally. "Are those Virginia Slims?"

"Indeed they are," he says. "Want one?"

I do, sort of. I need to make the best of this. I am in a bar with someone who is drinking vodka Slurpee, and I can't leave. I quit smoking last year but I feel a cigarette is in order here. When he's in the bathroom I get another Diet Coke and I ask for rum in it; I pay for it quickly before he gets back.

Terry is looking over at a girl at the table near the door. "See her? That girl is totally my type," he says. I have no idea what his type is, but she's pretty. "She wouldn't give me a second look, though." I don't know what to say to that.

He says, "I used to be so much better looking, like in my freshman year of college."

I don't know what to say to that either.

"Yeah, I used to be cute," he says. "When I was like, nineteen or twenty, twenty-one. I used to get hit on all the time."

I think he wants me to say something to sort of reassure him. He lights another Virginia Slim. I manage to say, "Wow."

He pours himself more Slurpee and orders another shot of Ketel One. Wow. It's nowhere near ten-thirty or even ten o'clock.

Now Terry is describing his "type" and then tells me to guess his favorite movie actress based on these specifications. "Girl-next-door type. Brunette. Come on."

I hate games like this and I'm never good at them.

"Come *on*. Career in the '60s. Big brown eyes."

"Natalie Wood," I answer.

"Yep. That's it. That's totally *it*," he says, grinning, pleased with himself. Though it's not like he was the one guessing.

We watch the TV some more. "So what about you?" he asks me.

"Like, what's my type?" I'm thinking it must be my turn to talk about this.

"No, I mean, okay: you would be really cute if you lost like, thirty pounds, you know?" He doesn't face me when he says this.

When I say "Oh, yeah?" I mean for it to sound different, but the thread of nerve in my voice seems to have slipped out and away.

"No, really, why don't you just lose thirty pounds?" he

asks. "You could have any guy in the bar if you lost twenty, thirty pounds." He offers me another cigarette.

"Whatever. I know," I'm saying. "Maybe I know that, okay?" I'm looking down at the cigarette I've taken and then at the pictures above the bar and anywhere that isn't to the immediate left where this guy is sitting.

"Well, I'm telling you. You could. Thirty pounds," he says. "Twenty. What's stopping you?"

He goes on talking. He knows how it is to gain a few pounds and all, he says. He says he knows it's hard to tell now, but he used to be way better looking, he used to get girls hitting on him all the time, and although he's told me all this before, he seems to have forgotten because he repeats himself verbatim. He sips some more vodka Slurpee. He says that back when he was better looking, he probably wouldn't have considered me in his league. "I know that sounds shallow?" he says. "But no. I wouldn't have gone for you. Unless you weighed a lot less, you know? Or I mean, a little less. Thirty pounds is really not a lot when you think about it. Why don't you lose thirty pounds?"

What I want to know is, why *thirty* pounds? He keeps coming back to that number. He says it so often I begin to wonder if he has some kind of secret knowledge. Thirty can't be arbitrary, can it?

"So why don't you? Come on," he says. Apparently he is waiting for a reasonable answer, as anyone drinking bright red eighty-proof slush naturally would be.

Part of me wants to just tell him that as a matter of fact I *have* been doing something, but then, I don't want his approval. I don't want to be a part of his personal science fair

ruled by types and leagues and distances measured in esti-
mated thirty-pound increments. I don't want to tell him
I've been doing Weight Watchers for the past four months.
In fact, I almost wish I wasn't doing it. I was more defiant
back when I was just fat, I think. I mean I'm not sure but I
think I would *have* to have been. Maybe twenty pounds
ago I had a better inner bitch, a snarky mastermind who
could navigate the rest of me, like that scene from *Aliens*
with Ripley in the powerloader, stomping around like a big
fat robot of justice and able to muster up the appropriate
response to a situation like this one. I should have been
able to shoot down Terry and his stupid femme cigarettes
and his ghetto daiquiri with powerful blasts of big-girl sass,
and also, lasers.

Instead, I just roll my eyes at him. It's all I seem to know
how to do. Roll my eyes as if they'll take me somewhere
else. I wonder if I will ever be thin enough to never have
another conversation like this.

"But you are thinking about it, right?" he says. "I can
tell you're thinking about doing it. You know if you lost a
few pounds you could get any guy you wanted. I wouldn't
say it if it wasn't true." All this time he has been talking to
my face by way of the flocked mirror tiles behind the bar;
I finally look over and see that he's been having the whole
conversation with this little scene of both of us.

He's still talking. "You know it's true, right?" he asks. I
look straight at him in the reflection and he nods at me as
if I've just joined him.

My drink isn't close enough to being done. I would like
him to go away. The bar noise that is behind the sound of

him talking, the TV and jukebox and the people at the pool table, it all needs to swell louder and close around this guy until he's submerged and gone. Not just his voice; all of him gone. I would like the background to obliterate him.

"You okay?" he asks me after I've turned back to the TV.

"I'm fine."

"What are you doing now?" he asks.

"I'm waiting for some friends."

"I got some DVDs tonight. I rented *Stagecoach*. You ever see that? You should see it."

"I saw it a long time ago."

"I'm right over here on Eastwood. We should pick up a six-pack and we'll watch it."

"Well, no. I'm meeting friends." I can't believe he is trying to get me to go home with him.

"No, you're not."

"Yeah, I think I am."

"They aren't coming. Come *on*."

"Oh, fuck you. They're at the Davis."

"*Okay*," he says. "But you know, if you change your mind"—he leans forward and points out the big window down the block to where he says his corner is—"I'm right over there. Do you see it?"

"Yes," I lie.

"I'm sorry if I, like, upset you before."

"I'm fine," I lie.

He has taken one of the little folding beer promotion signs that are at each table, and he's torn it open and he's writing his phone number on the blank side. His address, too, with instructions to Ring Bell for Hollis. He hands it to me.

"Here. I'm going to go home now and order some food. I'm gonna watch these movies. I got the classic John Fords. You should come by after you see your friends. We'll hang out."

It's a little after 10:30.

He says, "Think about what we were talking about, you know?"

He sets the box of Virginia Slims on the bar. "You want the rest of these?" he asks. Yes, I do. God fucking dammit. Then he's gone.

"You're *smoking*," says Leigh, when she and Richard find me.

"I'm ready to go somewhere else," I tell them.

domainatrix

We're sorry, but "pound.com" is not an available domain address. You may wish to consider:

pound.org

pound.tv

pound.biz

Click here to search for more options. Click here to search for similar domain names with the .com extension.

The following domains with the .com extension are still available:

beating.com

beatingdown.com

hammer.com

hammering.com

ram-down.com

rammed.com

rammed-down.com

ramming.com

ram-on.com

Click here to return to the main results page. Click here to search for available domains that contain "pound."

The following domains that contain "pound" are still available:

poundaround.com

pounded.com

poundinfo.com

poundopportunities.com

poundnow.com

poundtoday.com

poundworld.com

Click here to search for more options. Click here for a new domain name search.

Congratulations! The domain "poundy.com" is available. Click here to purchase the domain "poundy.com."

Are you sure you would like to purchase the following domain?

poundy.com

Click here to continue.

"Does Poundy.com sound like porn?" I ask Michael on the phone.

"I thought your site was called Pound," he says.

"I couldn't get it. I got *'Poundy'* instead. Does it sound bad?"

"Pound-EE? With a 'y?' Why'd you pick that?"

"I don't know. I wanted something close and it was all I could come up with. Does it sound like porn? Because you would know."

"Um, I only know gay porn."

"Okay. Your *limited* experience of porn notwithstanding, DOES IT SOUND LIKE PORN?"

"Why would it sound like porn?"

"Well," I think. "Like . . . *pounding*. Or, like, ramming. Except, not *ramming* but you know, pounding, I guess."

"Like with a *fist?*"

"Oh, God, no."

"It's okay. Poundy is fine."

"Are you sure?"

"Really."

Later he emails me: "I FOUND THIS NICE PICTURE ON THE INTERNET FOR YOUR POUNDY SITE. YOU LIKE?!" He's attached a JPEG file and when I open it it's every bit as disgusting as I've come to expect from Michael.

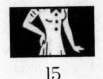

my self-esteem is none of your business

The first email that comes from a complete stranger is not unwelcome but it's mystifying enough that I save it in a folder I've named just "?". I don't really know what to do with it. Answer it? The woman was writing in response to an entry I posted last week where I described a day filled with totally Satanic food habits, eating hot buttered babies practically, and how much I loved it after having a perfect *POINTS!* regimen the day before, and does that make me a whore or what?

The subject line of this woman's email says *me, too.* She says she can completely relate and that her boyfriend calls her Fried Chicken Slut. She's signed her name Jenny.

Does she want me to be her friend? I wonder how this works.

I write her back: "What's up, Chicken Slut? Thanks for writing. I hope you keep reading! Best, Wendy." I hit SEND with a slight flutter of panic. I hope I wrote enough and that I didn't sound all self-aggrandizing with that "thanks for writing" stuff.

When I tell my friend Leigh about this she says, "She isn't going to show up at your house one day, is she?"

"She can't. She doesn't know my last name so she can't stalk me in person."

I say this but later it does occur to me that this Jenny person could keep emailing me. Or if not her, then some-one else, someone who might be more verifiably creepy. A person who maybe doesn't leave the house enough and who stays in chain-smoking and auctioning crumpled shirts and old extension cords on eBay. I mean I always wonder about the people who do stuff like that, and maybe one of them reads me. Maybe she bids on things that re-mind her of me. Maybe she is making a collage about me. Someone could just do that: make a collage and scan it and email it to me, and nobody could stop her.

As it turns out, Jenny doesn't write back, and I'm vaguely disappointed.

Almost all the emails are from women. Many of them mention Weight Watchers. They say they're on the pro-gram, too, or else they're thinking about doing it, or they've done it before and they're trying to get back on track.

I like hearing from them. A lot of them seem like me, but then I'm surprised at the differences. One woman has just gotten down to 265 pounds from around 310; another says she can finally fit back into her size 8 jeans again. Sometimes they have good stories of their own. A girl in San Francisco tells me that her Weight Watchers group meets in a Goth nightclub that rents out space during the day. I'm jealous that I don't get to tell that story, because there's a joke about fat girls wearing black in there somewhere.

They all remind me of people I've talked to on the CTA el and in airplanes, in conversations where the small talk stumbles into something bigger: everyone is in transit, in the middle of something. Everyone is changing themselves, or about to change, and reading my site is something they do in the meantime. There's a blurry quality to a lot of the exchanges since we don't really know each other. I want to write them all back; when I spend a whole night writing readers back it feels like time stands still.

There's a woman who has written me two or three times now telling me about her weight problems from having PCOS. I have to look up PCOS because I don't know how to ask her what it is. It stands for Polycystic Ovarian Syndrome. I don't write her back because I'm afraid of saying the wrong thing.

Someone named Sherilyn writes me and tells me she's lost forty-five pounds:

> *Sister, it's easy, you just eat less and burn more calories. I lost 45 lbs this way and also just by walking, have you tried the mall?*

She says that since I am in Chicago I should go to Woodfield Mall. She went there once while visiting a friend and it's big! She is under the impression that Woodfield Mall is an amazingly well-kept secret that has simply eluded me until now but at the same time is probably just down the street or something. She says I ought to go there at least two times a week, in the morning, and I should walk the mall four to six times, two to three times per level, and I can alternate directions and levels so I do not get bored. If I do this she can guarantee that I will lose at least thirty-five pounds.

Someone whose address is Phil Something at Earthlink but who signs his or her name "Mo" wants to know if I've tried the Atkins Diet, because even though he or she, Phil or Mo, has personally never tried it, he or she hears it works and maybe I should think about it.

Aeon Flux, not her real name I presume, says that even though I may not know it, I am beautiful. She can tell. I do not believe I have ever met Aeon Flux but she wants me to know that I am beautiful inside and she doesn't want me to be so full of hate, so full of loathing and shame for myself.

Someone named ~tweetye~ writes and says, simply:

> *dont do weightwatchers it sux. jenny craig is better*

I hit REPLY and type:

> *no way weight watchers rulZ!!!! jenny craig is a man i heard she has a dick!!!*

Twice I come close to clicking SEND before I finally just close the window and delete the thing. Anyone that profoundly estranged from the Shift key is not someone I want to mess with.

Usually it's good to get the emails but when it's not it's like AngelKara from the weight loss bulletin board has come back, hydra-headed and with a vengeance.

One night I find myself typing up a Frequently Asked Questions section:

Q: *Can I email you to tell you about the Atkins Diet? The Zone plan? Jenny Craig? Et cetera?*

A: No. Go away.

Q: *How much do you want to lose?*

A: Enough so that I can shop for clothes wherever the hell I want. Enough so that people don't presume that I have a goddamn character flaw and automatically give more credit to thin people, even the ones who shoplift, or tell crappy jokes, or believe in Scientology.

Q: *Is that so wrong?*

A: No.

Q: *So what is that in terms of pounds?*

A: Hell, I don't know.

Really, I don't.

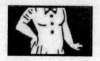

proof

"You're coming to my sister's wedding, right?" Leigh keeps asking me during her Saturday shift at Shucker's. By that she means: I'm driving out to Pennsylvania for at least a day and a half of righteous, all-expenses-paid drinking with her family, *right*?

Leigh Kendall has very blond eyelashes, which were very startling on her as a child. I saw this firsthand in third grade; she was a year younger and I knew her in passing as That Little Kid with the Space Eyes. She was wearing mascara in high school and we knew each other a little better then. Then in college, during holiday breaks and summers home, we became good friends. Often she'd drive us in her family's scratched-up Subaru to Toys "R" Us or Indiana for no reason at all. And we visited every restaurant we could find with the word *Golden* in the name, though we decided that Chinese restaurants didn't count, only all-night pancake houses with francheezies on the menu and fake stained-glass panels over the fluorescent light fixtures. There are more of these in northern Illinois than you might realize.

We did not have fake IDs. But then, hanging out at Leigh's house was like being an exchange student to a country called Grown-up Drinking, where Leigh's parents played the role of friendly host family graciously showing me the customs. I learned about gentle, sustained daytime drinking during their Fourth of July barbeques, and the Kendalls taught me about the better beers and how to play board games while buzzed on them. When they moved to Pennsylvania, Leigh and her big sister Kelly stayed behind in Chicago and found an apartment in my neighborhood. I sort of miss the Kendalls; I miss the age I was when they were around.

Now Leigh bartends at a seafood restaurant in the Gold Coast, a place that is dim inside and pricey, and when I visit her there these days I turn down free drinks because I am on Weight Watchers.

"I don't know if I can go," I tell her. I have work. I don't like leaving work sometimes. And I wonder what will happen if I leave my website behind for almost a week. I am afraid that I will forget everything I have learned so far about putting up web pages. One time I didn't update for three days, and I uploaded a page to the wrong folder, and I couldn't figure out why it wouldn't show up in my browser, and there was so much pain and sorrow, I swear. Leigh might not understand.

"You better come," she says.

"I know."

"They keep asking if you're coming. You know my mom always asks how you are. She says congratulations."

"About what?" I ask.

"I told her you lost fifteen pounds."

"You mean it's that big of a deal?"

"I know it kind of is for you," Leigh says. "I know you don't want it to be. But I mean, it's great."

"Yeah, I guess."

"After Stuart, you needed to do something like this," she says. "You know, for yourself."

Stuart is a regular here at Shucker's now, along with a handful of other people who Leigh used to serve drinks to at Barrett's before it closed last year. Barrett's was nice; it had strings of white lights crisscrossing the ceiling and the light flattered everyone. I don't like this place as much: I always find seafood restaurants to be sort of deathlike and bleak, what with all the dank blue in the color scheme, and the inevitable marlin trophy with the memory of its own final horror shellacked permanently in its eye. I was here with Stuart twice, and the second time, Leigh took me aside and informed me he was seeing someone behind my back.

But after Stuart I started going to therapy with Elizabeth. That was almost a year ago now. I remind Leigh of this.

"It's still good what you're doing, though," she says.

"It's not like an 'I Will Survive' kind of thing."

"Yes, and I'm pretty sure the DJ at Kelly's wedding won't play that, okay? Because you're coming. Right?"

"I just have to see about work." I'm always like this. It's only five days—three days and a weekend I'll be gone, but still.

I have been picking at the label of my Miller Lite bottle since even before I finished it. Leigh takes it and I let her get me one more drink before I go. It's late afternoon and a lot of her regulars come in with the dinner crowd, and I know better than to stay much longer.

Already Margaret has come in. Margaret is in her fifties and she has a husky laugh from smoking Tareytons, which I've never seen anyone else in the world buy. She says I look great. "Leigh says you're going to the big wedding," she says. I don't remember exactly when the Barrett's crowd began to feel like Leigh's extended family and people like Margaret got to be like crazy aunts and second cousins once removed. A few of them still tell me I am too good for Stuart.

"Take some pictures," she says to Leigh. "You have to bring back pictures of you girls all dressed up."

I tell her I'm not sure if I can go but I *probably* will. Leigh is nodding. Margaret says, "Oh, let yourself have some fun, right? You look good."

I think about it. I wonder if everyone wants me to have a *look-at-me-now* moment. Maybe I need to have one. It's hard to take any pride in being Too Good for Stuart, since all it really means is that I deserve better than a guy who wears a cell phone clipped to his belt and yells "Get a job!" at panhandlers. But to be *so* good that I became thinner just by not being with him is something else entirely. If I repel high-functioning alcoholics *and* unwanted pounds with the power of my goodness, I suppose I ought to let the world know. I'll get a nice dress and wear it as proof.

Leigh puts down a fresh cocktail napkin and sets a new drink on it. When I sip it the rum vapor hits my sinuses with a light *ping* and when I taste it I can tell it's made with Coke; there's real non-diet Coca-Cola in there.

"Holy shit." It's like drinking a cask of molasses with chaser swigs of rum. It's like drinking a whole fucking pirate ship. Rum and Coke is sort of a goofy drink, but I love it and I haven't had a real one in so long.

"You're coming to Pennsylvania," says Leigh.

xx girls

I guess I need a dress. For this there is Lincolnwood Town Center Mall. It has a Lane Bryant on the first floor, an Old Navy near the center junction, and a Carson, Pirie, Scott & Co. department store on the south end, where I park my car one night after work.

Carson's has a Misses Department, a Women's Department for plus sizes, and a Better Dresses Department. I walk around them wondering where I'd find a nice, sort of understated cocktail dress in around a size 18. Something black and a little fitted, I'm thinking.

Misses doesn't have anything formal enough; Better Dresses has one dress that's not bad but it's at least a size too small. The name *Better* Dresses implies that there are worse dresses somewhere and that's where Women's Studio comes in.

Women's Studio has a very limited display area: the one

mannequin is wearing some kind of awkward work ensem-
ble. There's a maroon cardigan layered over a maroon
turtleneck worn over a skirt with a muddy paisley print. I
know this look and I call it Repressed Woman with a Repressed Career. When I look closer I can see that the cardigan is actually fused to the sweater underneath. For some
reason, plus-size designers love the mutant conjoined twin-
set. I think they're under the impression that fat women
get so out of breath putting their arms through sleeves that
they're doing us a favor by simplifying things.

I shouldn't have come here. I know exactly what I will
find. Technically, it's a different Carson's at a different mall
from the one I shopped at with my mom when I was growing up, but really, it's the same place: the neutral lighting
is the same, the white melamine cashier counters, the
dressing rooms with whiffs of starch, with no room to stand
back and see what you're wearing from a safe distance.

It doesn't feel like the clothes are much different. An
alarming number of the dresses here have Auntie Mame
touches like sequins, and animal prints, and floaty sleeves.
Also, what I call the I'm-Chubby-But-Huggable look is big
here: there are novelty sweatshirts with *things* on them in
scary, crusty formations; puffy acrylic designs and clouds
and animal faces.

There are almost never sales ladies around in the
Women's Studio area. There's a service counter but it's
usually empty. If you buy something you have to go across
the aisle to the Petites section. The way the clothes for
large women are right next to the clothes for small women
has a creepy circus logic to it that I could appreciate more

if they had a department for all the other sideshow women. They'd have special carny jeans with three legs, sweaters with extra-small turtlenecks for the pinheads, stuff like that. I'd love to see that.

Next is Lane Bryant.

Liv Tyler's sister is so pretty. She's on a poster in the window of Lane Bryant. She wears the Lane Bryant jeans with high heels, and she stands there, arms akimbo, being defiantly Not-Her-Skinny-Sister. I think the family resemblance and the slight sting of comparison is what makes Mia Tyler such a great plus-size model and so perfect for the Lane Bryant stores. The whole idea is that Lane Bryant understands how you feel: you bring your fat girl pain to Lane.

Lane Bryants strive to look like classy boutiques, like the sort of place where you stride through with a bouquet of shopping bags and a pillbox hat and a sense of purpose. Their very generous fitting rooms with wide, stylish veneer doors convey Big Girl Entitlement. All in all, Lane Bryant does a very convincing job at being a mall store. I've heard that thin girls will sometimes walk into Lane Bryant and for the longest time have no idea where they are.

The salesgirl working the floor says, "Hi, welcome to Lane Bryant."

"I know," I say.

I've shopped at Lane Bryant long enough that I can look at the other women shopping in the store and pick out the Lane Bryant clothes they happen to be wearing that day. There is a woman poking through the jean shelves who's wearing one of the duster sweaters that I tried on last fall but didn't buy; the salesgirl is wearing a wrap blouse that I own in a different color. Every now and then I used to say "Oh, I have that, *too*!" to the women who work at Lane Bryant until I realized that they probably hear that all day long.

Really, everyone shops at Lane Bryant if they're larger than a size 16. There are other plus-size store chains, but Lane Bryant's stuff most closely approximates whatever the rest of the world is wearing. You really have to be impressed with their efforts. Today while I'm browsing, I can tell Lane Bryant really wants me to know they're very aware of the current folksy trend: the peasant blouse. They're *on* it. They've whipped up a big batch of peasant style *just for us*.

There is only one black dress at Lane Bryant today and the closest size in stock is a 20. It's okay. It's sort of big, but it's okay, though it's loose, has slippery "illusion" fabric sleeves, and it wasn't really what I was looking for.

I try one of the peasant blouses on. I phone Richard from the fitting room.

"Yeah, so I look like a fucking Renaissance fair right now."

"Bite my turkey leg, baby," he says.

I leave the fitting room and walk around carrying the black dress while I look at other things. The sleeves keep sliding off the plastic hanger and I guess if I really liked it I would be making more of an effort to fix it.

A different salesgirl stops me. "Would you like to try that on?"

I did. But I guess I will again.

The dress really is not good. It has a high empire waist that makes me look like I'm either knocked up or an adult ward of the state. It balloons out a little. It doesn't look any better when I take off my wool socks. I wish I could see how it looks in my own size but I'm pretty sure it wouldn't be an improvement. It's not awful in any empirical way, but it's still clearly a mistake. It makes me look like I don't understand myself.

I hate to admit the dress is wrong because I'm at Lane Bryant and they're trying so hard. When I'm in Lane Bryant and there's nothing I like there, I feel a little like the universe has failed me, though I guess, really, it's an alternate universe, a slightly compromised one where you have to go around thinking, really, it's all right until some evidence to the contrary totally betrays you. My friend Colette Molloy's parents only let her listen to Christian rock and she must have felt this way sometimes.

I feel like this even though I know I don't have to shop mostly at Lane Bryant anymore. I don't have to stay here; I'm a size smaller now, and I can slip out and escape. And that's what I do.

Old Navy has clothes for women up to size 20 and down to size 2 or maybe even 0. They also have stuff for men, and kids, and infants; they're so exuberantly inclusive you almost can't stand it; there's a brassy, theme-park feel to their Everybodyness. One time I wandered over to a very cute accessory display near the entrance and had been staring at it in my appreciative retail trance for at least a full

minute before I realized I was looking at stuff for dogs—
travel bowls and toys and collars and cunning little ban-
dannas, because hell, why not have dogs be part of the
damn parade.

It's dumb, but I like this place. It's still sort of new to
me. After I lost about ten pounds I figured out I could shop
here, and when I first walked in I felt like I'd finally found
the place where they hand out the normal clothes to the
normal people. I felt like I'd joined the world. I mean when
I come here it feels official somehow, like I am reporting
for assignment in the ranks of the big bright fashion Here
and Now. Go destiny! Go track pants! Over the sound system they play a song I used to roller skate to, I think.

They have dresses in the front, and more dresses stuffed
in the back, and some are even folded and wedged onto
shelves. I grab stuff in 16s and 18s and 20s and XLs and Ls
and XXLs; multiple sizes of the same thing and then pre-
cious single items that I find all by themselves, in just the
one size that might fit. When it's busy at Old Navy there's
a cheerful hell-has-broken-loose spirit to things; the whole
place looks a bit like a stockroom that one is encouraged
to raid.

None of the things I pick out are right for a wedding
but I'm trying them on anyway because Old Navy
Women's XXL is the only thing that fits me. It is somewhere just above a women's 14–16, which makes it, in
truth, an XL with an extraneous X. I've thought about this
a lot. Xs are not exponential: XXL is not twice the X of XL.
Rather, XX = X + 1. As I leave the fitting rooms, my ears
are sort of ringing from the music, and the kids who work

here keep talking on their headsets and exchanging blasts of static. All that is known of X is that it means there's always more: it makes something out of nothing. Therefore, having to wear an X size ought to mean nothing to me, though of course it doesn't.

I have to go back through Carson's to get back to my car. I don't know why I stop at Women's Studio again. Compared with the other stores it's dim; it's quiet enough to hear the hum of the heating system.

I started coming here by myself in high school and I remember sometimes I wouldn't even try the other stores first. There's a weird, furtive comfort to shuffling through the hangers and I sort of feel it even now. I guess when I'm looking for something, it's just my nature to go back to the first place I searched. So I come back here, and the clothes aren't mine, and eventually I decide nothing's missing.

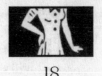

third eye

I was in sixth grade when *Young Miss* magazine began appearing in the mail. Our mail came in through a big brass slot; the postal carrier fed it through in big bundles that would hit the floor of our enclosed front porch and scatter on impact. Every afternoon brought a fresh new postal explosion. One day my mom picked through the debris and handed something to me. "I guess this is for you," she said. It was a copy of *Young Miss*. The paper label in the corner showed that it was addressed to me, but of course it couldn't have been for anyone else in our household. I was sort of flattered to be singled out for my youthful missyness in this way, but nobody had any idea how the magazine had come to me. "Maybe you got on some mailing list somewhere," my mom said. Really it felt as if the universe had suddenly recognized me and sent me a summons of some kind.

I flipped through the pages. There were stories and photos and kicky graphic-design squiggles. There were *ads*: Bonne Bell and Tampax and Goody barrettes. They looked almost like adult ads. It felt oddly satisfying to see things being marketed to me without cartoon characters.

I took the magazine over to the couch and started reading it. Mostly I enjoyed it. I can't say *Young Miss* actually excited me; instead, it had a certain equable quality to it which seemed to have something to do with all the things the magazine *didn't* have. It was blissfully free of puzzles and riddles and "discussion questions." It was definitely more aloof than *The Weekly Reader* most of the time, but then it was also startlingly friendly enough to include a regular feature called "Was My Face Red!" where readers shared mortifying true stories about their underwear and/or feminine hygiene products peeking out of their clothes, or falling out of their gym bags, or otherwise emerging at the worst fucking possible moment ever.

I read the whole issue carefully. Then the next month *Young Miss* showed up in the mail again, like a sign of approval.

The covers of *Young Miss* always featured a girl who appeared to be a couple of years older than me. But she wasn't so old that I could get away with not paying attention to her, the way I'd only semiconsciously skimmed grown-up glam in my mom's Avon catalogs. She was just old enough that when I looked at her I felt obligated to notice the details—the lip gloss and the plastic earrings; the ponytail to one side. I remember one cover girl wore a braided headband that went straight across her forehead.

Designer headbands like that were hot accessories, and I wanted one badly; wanted to wear it through the portal of 1983 into the dazzling New Wave future. But my sixth grade teacher, Ms. Belisonzi, did not approve of them because she said they covered our "third eyes." These, she said, were in the middle of our forehead and they helped us sense things we couldn't see otherwise.

Although I wasn't in junior high yet, I had an exercise regimen. Or I did for a little while at least, in the summer after sixth grade. For years after it remained the most conscientious routine I'd ever had.

I'd wake up and ride my bicycle. They'd just put down blacktop in the neighborhood and I pedaled in the weekday morning quiet, learning to work the gears of my mom's abandoned three-speed, listening to them tick down whenever I slowed. The way an adult bicycle could glide on such thin tires was sublime to me, but while I loved the ride, I couldn't quite bring myself to ride freely and without a routine. Mentally, I'd plot out a route around the blocks—three short blocks, turn; two long blocks, turn; and I'd circle around.

It was late June and my parents were at work and the days had nothing in them, and I rode long enough to wear a groove into the surface of every day.

I remember coming back inside after the ride and eating half a container of Yoplait cherry yogurt, saving the rest for the next day. I probably remember these things so well because that was the part I mastered: I gave myself things to do right and I did them.

My mom noticed the opened containers of yogurt in the fridge and asked me if I was dieting. I knew that since she was a therapist that when she asked something like that it was a Serious Thing.

"No," I told her. It was mostly true; I still went to Mc-Donald's; I lined up for pizza at the block party. "I'm just watching things," I said.

My sixth grade class was pretty indignant over the Third Eye Issue. Whenever Ms. Belisonzi mentioned it we'd be all, *No way! We so do not have another EYEBALL somewhere!*

"Sure you do," Ms. Belisonzi would say. She had Greenpeace stickers stuck to her desk; most of our science units were about endangered species. She dressed in L.L. Bean corduroy skirts and cotton turtlenecks, and every one of her pendant gemstone necklaces had its own story of origin, though I can't remember any of us ever asking her to tell us. "The third eye helps with perception. It's like an invisible eye."

An invisible eye? we'd howl.

"An invisible eye. You can't see it, but it's there."

We'd really get fed up at this point: protesting, rolling our actual, legitimate eyes, and making the sort of exasperated, snorting sighs that only the Young and The Fucked With can pull off. They were pretty much the same noises we made at Halloween when we found out the only candy at our class party would be raisins, raisins coated with carob.

But aside from all the New Age controversy, the matter

of the designer headbands was really only the girls' problem. Kara Tessler and Joo Yun Jung would slip theirs on
when we went to Mrs. Smitherman's room for Social Studies on Tuesdays and Thursdays. They were two of the most
popular girls in class and having to constantly take their
headpieces off and put them on again gave them a bizarre
kind of authority, like queens in exile.

Once, Stephanie LeBeau came to class with a new
headband. She was by far the tallest in the class; a black,
mawkishly sweet girl with such a soft voice that nobody
ever gave her much trouble. Everyone seemed to sense her
discomfort at being so tall even as we suspected she could
kick ass, too. She got to wear her headband all day, but she
tripped on her way to the pencil sharpener. Her gym shoes
squeaked on the tile and she almost fell down altogether.
"*See?*" said Ms. Belisonzi. "See what happens?"

Young Miss had a thing for doing fashion spreads without
people. They liked to lay out clothes and accessories in
paper doll fashion to form complete outfits—beret on top,
ankle boots on bottom. Flat sleeves and jean legs were bent
to form various jaunty poses; they looked just fine without
a body. I was never quite convinced that any of the clothes
could dress me up even half as well as they did the white
space of the page in *Young Miss*.

It was one thing to look at the models in some of the
other fashion layouts of the magazine. A group of them
horsed around prettily in a back-to-school style feature:
caught in midair jumping over a pile of leaves; balancing
on the top step of a set of bleachers; vamping studiously

with old books used as props. Their first names ran along-side their pictures so that we'd get to know them: there was Tracey, and Kirsten, and even Whitney, who went on to become Whitney Houston, God help her. These girls I could survey from a distance; if I wanted to consider them friends, or sisterly fashion mentors, or credit them with all the "Was My Face Red!" stories that involved inadvertent, public, and totally time-stopping thunderclap farts, it was up to me. I could play along from a distance.

But it was another thing entirely to look at the empty clothes. It felt as if *Young Miss* was handing the assembly instructions off to me, laying out all the parts I'd need to be the Best Me Possible, but I still didn't understand how they all fit together. And I wasn't sure they'd fit *me*.

I don't actually remember what my body looked like or how much I weighed during the summer I rode my bicycle around in the mornings. The pictures I have seem to indicate that I was overwhelmed by my breasts. I had a stretchy tube top that behaved in ways that can only be called passive-aggressive. I'm not really fat in any of the photos from that summer, but I can see that everything was a little too small—riding up, straining against me; there were straps that constantly needed to be straightened and adjusted.

I must have thought I needed vigilance. I must have thought this was the beginning of everything.

My mother had just lost eighty pounds as a result of her surgery. More than once some adult friend or family member would ask me "Are you glad your mother lost all that weight?" They must have been asking me if I was happy for her but to me it sounded like the question was, Wasn't I relieved? As if some kind of disaster had been averted.

Later that summer our family took a car trip to New Mexico; we went camping and made stops to visit family and old neighbors—it was on this trip that my mom posed for the picture with my great-aunt at the scenic overlook in Arkansas. Our station wagon would pull into strange driveways and people we knew would come out and greet us. They hadn't seen us in years, and invariably the first thing they'd say was to my mom: *You've lost so much weight*. The second thing they'd say to me: *You're growing up*.

Somehow my mother had made it back from weighing well over three hundred pounds: it took two surgeries, and after that, half a dozen hospital visits for complications; and before that, a succession of diet plans going back as far as I could remember. The shitty bricks-and-boards bookcase on the landing of our house held a row of obsolete weight-loss guides. There were pocket paperbacks of *The Scarsdale Diet* and the *Woman Doctor's Diet for Women*, as well as a handful of booklets picked up at the supermarket: calorie guides, carbohydrate counters, special recipes. For my mother, it amounted to a history of trial and error, but for me it felt like an opportunity. Already I knew that it was hard work to keep weight off but I was ready to do my job. There was no reason, I thought, why I shouldn't do well at it. In fact, maybe I was a prodigy. I took two Gifted and Talented Youth classes at the community college; I wanted to be smart enough to keep from getting fat.

It was all right there in one book or another: you could fill gallon jugs with water and use them as free weights. You could eat a hamburger without the bun. You could get off the bus a stop early and walk an extra three blocks every day for as many days as it took to not be fat.

I strove for that—that *not being*—much more than I did actual thinness. It was better that way, less confusing. From reading *Young Miss*, I knew better than to blatantly want to be popular or well-dressed, but I couldn't quite get the hang of Just Being, either, which was a sort of vague philosophy they endorsed in the kicky copy of their advice sections: i.e., Just Be Yourself. Rather than put on too much makeup, you could *just* dab on gloss and concealer; instead of dressing up in a flashy miniskirt to go to a movie, you could *just* put on your favorite chinos and go! Okay, but what the hell were *chinos*, I wondered, and was I supposed to have more than one and pick a favorite or what? Just Being was uncomfortable: it was like thinking about the spot in the middle of my forehead and feeling like something ought to be there, almost an itch.

Once or twice I decided to ride block after block as long as I could, just to see when I'd be overcome with the feeling of wanting to turn back. The side streets were empty and sedate enough that I could make a U-turn when the impulse hit, and my energy felt like a long cord that grew taut once I'd reached the end of it. Each time I turned back I felt I hadn't gone far enough, but the burning in my legs discouraged me from trying again the next day, and I went back to counting street blocks.

I don't remember if I lost any weight. I don't remember why I stopped. I know at some point the weather changed.

The *Young Miss* magazines kept coming all year. Sometimes when I got them I felt a little like I was getting away with something.

That Thanksgiving my grandmother looked at me and said, "Do you know I forgot to tell you that I got you a subscription to some teen magazine? It was months and months ago when I did it, with that Publishers Clearing House thing. Did you ever get it? You got it, right?"

#

every day is a gift

The fantasy is a single scene in which I run into an acquaintance who hasn't seen me in a while, during which time I have lost fifty pounds.

"*Hey* there!" Acquaintance says. "*Hi!*" We are passing each other on the street and the surprised lilt in his voice is a little hook that tugs us both into stopping.

I said *his*, right? Let's say this is a guy. Acquaintance is quite often a guy in this.

"Is that you? You look *great!*" he says. I shrug, sort of embarrassed. "No, really!" Acquaintance says. "I almost didn't recognize you! Wow!"

I change the subject, of course.

We ask each other what we've been up to lately. My answers are vague. Acquaintance's answers are unimportant, although he may report that he has broken up with his most recent girlfriend, who may or may not be one of those exceedingly petite girls who wear daft little thrift-store tees and plastic spider jewelry to play up her cunning, offbeat sexiness. Which is not to say I'm irritated by shit like that. No, not here. I have other things to think about.

Acquaintance goes on talking for a couple minutes while I nod politely. Then he asks me if he can call me sometime.

"Well." I look away. "I don't know . . . maybe. I don't know. Long story," I say.

"You'll have to tell me sometime." Acquaintance smiles. "Seriously. You look great these days. Really *good*."

"Really?" I ask.

"Oh, yeah," he says.

Here is where I get to say it.

I say, "Fuck you! I had cancer!"

The guy's smile collapses like sand.

"*That's* why I'm so damn thin! I had *cancer*, okay?"

He's stunned. He tries to apologize.

"No . . . just . . . forget it," I say in disgust.

He opens his mouth to say something, but then stops himself. He is bewildered by his own gall, he is almost choking on it in fact.

Maybe I tremble a little, because I'm still weak. Or I nervously reach up to fix my hair, because suddenly I have a wig on. There's a wig sometimes, or one of those stocking caps that are, you know, all cute. With great weariness in my voice I tell Acquaintance about my harrowing battle with Type 3 Pseudokemia, and how it caused me to nearly wither away.

But I'm fine now, I tell him. Every day is a gift, I say.

to camelot

For the road trip to Pennsylvania I am packing a Special Bag with fruit and bottled water and popcorn cakes and *Just Two Points!* bars, which are clever little low-fat snack bars; they are like the Mormon cousins of candy bars.

I am taking my special book, *Weight Watchers Fast Food Companion*, which tells you how many *POINTS!* are in the food at more than two dozen fast-food restaurants. It's very informative. Sometimes I flip through it just for fun to see what the worst possible things I can eat are. A Dairy Queen Chicken Strip Basket with Texas Toast is twenty-three points. Think of the tragedy of getting your ass kicked at Dairy Queen like that without even eating ice cream.

I am becoming increasingly aware of the way hidden calories, like radiation, can taint the most innocuous things. Lately my Weight Watchers meetings have been full of all kinds of urban diet legends such as The Lady Who Used Too Much Butter Flavor Cooking Spray (Zero points per serving, the label said! She didn't know a whole can has *fifty points*! Dear God she *didn't know*!) and The Low-Fat Ice Cream Novelty Whose Manufacturer Changed The Recipe (It's not so low-fat anymore! How could we have *been so blind?!*). In each instance the moral is pretty much the same: some things are too good to be true, and we trust too much, and Soylent Green is people.

At my last meeting the topic was Fast Food Salad Dressings, which reportedly harbor secret fat calories the way doorknobs carry fecal matter. I noticed one woman had her hands clamped to the side of her head, just like in Edvard Munch's *The Scream*. I made fun of her on my website, but all the same, I'm taking the damn book.

I am packing a black dress that I found in a catalog. I ordered a size 18 and held my breath for the ten days it took to arrive and then sucked it in even more when I pulled it over my head for the first time.

It fit. A part of me feels it shouldn't have fit. I told Elizabeth that in our last session, just in case she thought everything was perfect with me.

I am also taking along Richard and his boyfriend, Nicholas, since they needed a ride. I have a feeling this is going to be a fun trip. Hence the need for the Special Bag.

I pick up Nicholas and Richard and while they're putting their stuff in the trunk I point out the Bag, sort of proudly.

"Uh, that's . . . *nice*," Nicholas says, delicately, as if I had taken up latchhooking or some other craft.

"Shut up, I need it." I think it's true: I need to be this much of a geek.

"Wow, so you're really doing this," Richard says.

"I've *been* doing it," I tell him. "I still am." Though I don't say I keep having to do it in bigger doses so that it continues to make sense.

We're taking the Chicago Skyway out. The road vaults up to the Skyway bridge that takes us over Calumet City, over barges and water treatment plants and electrical towers and big tanks of God knows what. We have to roll up the windows when we cross over into Indiana, through Hammond and Gary. The first hour of any trip east from Chicago takes you through panoramic swaths of industrial stuff, all of it ugly, all hell, and we love it. It makes Indiana into an epic.

"Let me try one of those candy bars," Nicholas says. He means the *Just Two Points!* bars. I have one in my purse and I let him find it while I drive. I glance over to see him taking a bite and then I turn back to the road. I glance over again and he's chewing.

I glance again: still chewing. He looks a little concerned. I look back at the road and pass another car.

When I look back Nicholas is nodding at me as if to say *still chewing*. Then he finishes chewing. He swallows.

"Thanks. That was interesting. You can have the rest of it."

We need to stop somewhere. It's been over two hours and we're starting to pay attention to billboards and to the fast-food logos on exit signs.

"Oh my God, Hardee's," Richard shouts from the back seat. "Have you ever been to a Hardee's?"

I know Richard has some kind of secret heavy metal past in Michigan and from the tone of his voice I can tell that Hardee's restaurants are some important part of that lost era. He actually presses himself against the car window as we pass the sign.

"Is it in the book?" I ask. My rule is that we can stop anywhere as long as it's in the *Weight Watchers Fast Food Companion.*

Nicholas flips through the pages. "It's in the book all right."

In the mirror I can see Richard's arm punch the air.

Hardee's is the next exit.

When you open the *Fast Food Companion* to page seventy-one, devoted to all things Hardee's, organ arpeggios start playing and the pages burst into flame.

"What's wrong?" says Nicholas. We're in the restaurant and Richard is already at the counter.

I show him where it says a Monster Burger is worth twenty-eight Weight Watcher points.

"Because it's a *Monster* Burger," he says. Nicholas is very sensible. "That's its *nature.*" He has a point.

A jumbo serving of Crispy Curls Potatoes (Jumbo! They say *jumbo* here!) is fourteen points. So is a Chicken Biscuit. I figure out it's possible to eat two whole days' worth of points in a single Hardee's meal, not including the time spent passed out in the food coma afterward. I can't stop doing perverse food math.

I get a ham and cheese sandwich, which is seven points. It's not bad. I can tell it's the same ham they pile on top of one of their fried chicken fillet sandwich selections. I guess ham is kind of like a condiment at Hardee's.

Richard gets a piece of fried chicken *and* a Frisco Burger: nine plus eighteen.

"*What?* I like Hardee's," Richard says.

We stop to switch drivers at a truck stop an hour from Ohio. Nicholas leaves a toiletries bag there. He'd gone to the rest room to take out his contacts and when he came out he left the bag on top of one of the waste bins.

"We can try and get it on the way back," I tell him.

"That's okay. I'm not going to go back and say 'Excuse me, do you have my *big faggy bag of man cosmetics?*'"

"Yeah, maybe not."

"What's a *wall drug?*" Richard asks.

"What?"

"It was on a bumper sticker. We passed it."

"Did it say, HAVE YOU DUG WAL-DRUG? That's some tourist stop in, like, South Dakota or something."

"So it's not a drug?"

"No, honey, I'm sorry."

Who knows all the lyrics to "The Real Slim Shady?" *Richard.*

*   *   *

Interstate 80 through Ohio has big shiny new rest stops; round, modern glass buildings that are like mall food courts dropped in the middle of farmland, huge friendly mother-ships. I don't even need the book. There is a fancy upscale sandwich place that serves salads.

The sun is getting low and it comes through the atrium windows. Having the sun glaring in the rearview mirror has been wearing us out slowly, but it's nice in here. More than we'd care to admit, we like that all the surfaces are wiped down, and all the telephones work, and everything is handicapped-accessible. I like that I can get a salad. Everything is very well-intentioned here.

I have to wait a long time for my salad to be made. Nicholas and Richard finish their sandwiches and watch me eat.

"That's a nice salad."

"It *is* a nice salad.

"You look great," says Richard, as if he is sorry about the salad.

We have to stop for the night eventually, and Columbus looks good. At the rest stop we'd stared at a big map under Plexiglas, dotted with logos of chain motels.

We try checking into a TraveLodge on the outskirts of Columbus but they're booked. It's after nine on a Friday. "Most places around here are booked by now," the clerk says. "The franchise places, at least."

Back in the car Nicholas says, "We don't have to stay

at one of the chain motels, do we? There're local places, right?"

"That might be fun," I say. I'm thinking of some vintage place with cabins. Cabins and a big old-fashioned neon sign.

Who accidentally stuck their big honking dress shoes on top of my Special Bag, smooshing everything? *Nicholas*.

The only neon on The Camelot Inn sign is the word VA-CANCY, but it gets kitsch credit for having Old English lettering running down the side of a miniature turret.

"I wonder if it has theme rooms," says Richard, though as we pull in we can see that aside from the goofy sign, the place is just like any aging motel—battered doors that face the parking lot, little windows, vinyl curtain linings facing out.

Nicholas and I go to the front office to check in. It's a small room with a Plexiglas window like a ticket booth. There is a clock radio and ashtrays and fluorescent light. The Plexiglas has all kinds of things stuck to it—Xeroxed signs: CHECK OUT TIME 10:00 AM OR CHARGED ANOTHER DAY and QUIET AFTER 11 PM WE CALL POLICE; charge card and travel club stickers; phone numbers for CAB and TOW typed on index cards; bounced checks with the names on them circled emphatically; a handwritten note that says, "Curtis Wayne Harris and Bobby Ray are not al-lowed on these premises;" a big neon sticker for a security company. The man in the booth has big glasses and looks like he belongs there. Before we can ask him anything we have to write down the model and license of my car on a grimy clipboard he pushes through the slot at us.

The key he gives us is big, like an old car key, and doesn't come on a ring.

"What number is it?" Nicholas asks. It's not on the key.

The manager pushes over a slip of paper that says *14*.

"Fourteen," says Nicholas, holding the key a little bit like it's dead.

"Go out and up the stairs," the manager says.

Nicholas hands me the key and I hold it gingerly, too.

Nicholas and Richard and I go along the open walkway until we get to the door. The first thing we notice about the room is that one of the beds seems to be falling down, or else the headboard that's bolted to the wall has come loose at one corner.

"Whose head did *that?*" I wonder aloud.

"I hope she got a good tip," says Richard.

The TV doesn't have a switcher knob, only a short metal stump, and there is a pair of pliers on the TV stand for that purpose, or so we hope that's the purpose.

There are cigarette burns everywhere. They are on the furniture, on the black plastic of the TV cabinet, in the drapes, and on the pleated lampshade of one of the little side table lamps. We think those dark marks on the ceiling are cigarette burns, even though we know this is crazy.

There's just the one lock and the chain latch. Our instinct is to use the chair, too, the sad little armchair. Richard takes it and tilts it so as to prop it under the doorknob. We can see the wood on the back of the chair is worn away exactly where everyone else did the same thing.

Richard goes into the bathroom. Nicholas and I are trying to figure out the TV. We're talking in hushed tones.

"This is *way* more than . . ." he starts.

"Yeah."

Nicholas is looking at the wall behind me. I look and see black scuff marks high up, as if shoes had been thrown at it.

"It's . . . wow."

"*Yeah.*"

"You guys?" Richard calls from the bathroom. "Uh, could you come in here for a minute?"

Richard is staring down at the toilet. There are two of the biggest condoms we've ever seen in our lives floating there.

Nicholas chokes and gasps and laughs all at the same time.

There's a cigarette burn in the shower curtain, too.

Bob Evans Restaurants are not in the *Fast Food Companion.* Bob Evans is a *family restaurant;* it has grandmotherly wallpaper and lacy curtains and it's musty with syrup smells and after-church atmosphere, even though it's not even Sunday. However it's just what we need after our night at the Camelot. A trailerless truck cab idled in the parking lot for well over an hour until around 2 A.M. We need coffee. "I was *semi*conscious all night," jokes Nicholas. "Sorry," he adds.

We slept with a lot of clothes on—sweatpants, socks,

T-shirts and everything, even though it's May. We weren't thinking about why; it just felt right. After what we saw in that bathroom we're pronouncing *Camelot* with a long *a* now.

Richard and Nicholas order big breakfast skillets with side orders of pancakes and meat, lots of Bob Evans's meat.

The Weight Watchers materials tell you to *mentally rehearse* situations. For example, if you are at a dinner and you know your host will offer you a second helping, you're encouraged to visualize yourself saying, *No thank you, the meal was absolutely delicious and I'm quite satisfied.* They actually call this *storyboarding.* You are supposed to imagine a desired outcome in your life through a series of panels, much like a storyboard for a film—or maybe a scene from a film, or a short film, or even a trailer, like a commercial for *How I Achieved My Sensible Yet Empowering Weight Loss!*, starring you.

I think the idea is that the story is supposed to make sense. It wouldn't be Bergmanesque and weird the way I think my little fake movie probably is. I think there's one panel where I'm trying on the black dress, another where I'm looking in the fucking book, then another where I'm not in the scene at all, where it's just what I'm looking at, which yesterday was the highway and the land on either side and the clouds and everything I kept trying to overtake in my car.

Then another scene where I'm on a cargo plane that never leaves the runway even though the engines are going. That would be from the dream I had last night, thanks to the idling truck outside the Camelot. Then finally me here.

The waitress brings me a plate that's as big as the ones she sets down in front of Nicholas and Richard.

"That looks good," Nicholas says. It is. It's the desired outcome: pancakes.

Richard has this idea that the people who left the giant condoms in our room at the *Camelot* are still in the area.

"Maybe they're here," he says,

"At *Bob Evans?*" asks Nicholas.

Richard points to a table nearby: two couples, eating breakfast. They are most definitely retired people. "It's *those* guys," he whispers.

it's raining men

Kelly Kendall and Bill We Forget His Name But Really He's The Best Guy Ever are married the day after we get to Pennsylvania. It's a sweet ceremony: the men in the wedding party wear kilts; the pastor makes gentle jokes; a guy with a bagpipe plays "Amazing Grace" just outside the church where it actually sounds wonderful (Bill We Forget His Name has a *Scottish* name, we know that much). When the wedding party files out we can see Leigh taking deep breaths every time the shuffling procession slows down, and she appears to be sort of choking the end of her bridesmaid bouquet. Leigh needs a cigarette. When we went to see *Titanic* Leigh wanted to wear a nicotine patch to get her through the three hours.

We stop back at our Holiday Inn room after the ceremony.

"Do I look okay?" I keep wanting to change my nylons.

They are Nude Tone though I don't know whose nudity they're trying to simulate. It does not appear to be mine. "Should I wear black nylons?"

"Why?" Nicholas asks.

"Well, because then that way with the black dress I create, you know, a longer line. Like a single line. Or something." I'm standing in the mirror gesturing up and down like a flight attendant giving safety instructions.

"Oh, shut up," Richard says. "You're not a line."

"Yeah, no kidding," I say. I look at my stomach.

"No, I'm serious," says Richard. "You've been working really hard, you know? You haven't been doing all this to be a fucking *line*."

The reception is in the Kendalls' big backyard in a rural subdivision. There's a tent with a dance floor, a buffet, a bar table by the garage. I hug Mr. and Mrs. Kendall and I want to bring them a great many cocktails. Richard and Leigh have claimed the side yard deck for the Republic of Smoking, and Bill the groom keeps glancing over in their direction. "Aw, *man*," he says.

"I'm sorry," I tell him. Kelly says he's quit, or he's trying to, at least. I barely know him but I like that he's trying today, of all days.

"Now, you're gonna go and say hi to my Tennessee boys, right?" he says. Bill is from around Knoxville and when he speaks his vowels are gently skewed. "They drove up here and they don't know anyone. You might want to talk to Peter." He points across the yard at a sleepy-eyed guy in a groomsman's kilt.

*   *   *

I think I thought the people I'd see here would be other people. This occurs to me after I start my second drink and feel the alcohol working like a ballast. Some part of me had thought Stuart would be here. It was never a possibility but nevertheless I'd half conjured him, along with trace expectations of random other people: people I knew in college, teachers, movie characters. When I went to my high school reunion I felt this way, too. I'd walked in and thought: *Oh, it's just you guys.* There was no story, not one that I was in, at least. It's like this now.

The wedding photographer comes by and I let him take my picture. He directs me to go over by a flower bed, and he waits until I find the right way to stand. When he's done he walks off and suddenly I'm a little bereft that the picture's stuck in the camera and I can't see how it turns out.

The familiar people who are here include the Kendalls' old neighbors in Oak Park, two of Leigh's less soggy regulars from Shuckers, and Evelyn Capaldi. Evelyn Capaldi I remember from high school: she was in the same class as Kelly Kendall, two years ahead of me. She was a theater person, though I had never seen her in a play. Now she is across the yard talking to two of the groomsmen.

Leigh looks over to where she is. "You know Evelyn, right?"

I do, sort of. I remember being at a cast party from one of the musicals, and there was Evelyn Capaldi in the living room by the piano, singing torchy renditions of all the lead solos. It might have been more than one party that I remember, but whatever the case, Evelyn was singing. What I remember most is that Evelyn was nearly 300 pounds. She still is.

Also, in 1987 she had a floral tapestry jacket. I don't know why this sticks out for me. Actually, I do: it's because she was fat—*fat*, not just ambiguously plump, but big, with the generous bosom and the full face, and the legs that tapered down to her pointy-toed flats in a way that was sort of exquisite even as it emphasized her size. I didn't quite understand how it was that she was fat but also had something I wanted. In high school I tended to avoid girls who were heavier than I. But then Evelyn Capaldi's tapestry jacket made her look cultured, like stylish artsyness permeated her everyday existence; she carried herself like she had already *arrived*.

"I'm writing a musical," I overheard her telling someone once. Then she broke into a song from it.

In high school my response to people like Evelyn Capaldi was simply to be shy: this way I could buy in to her schtick but reserve the option to see it for what it was. I did this with boys I liked and also with the pagan girl at my lunch table who claimed to be possessed; she was difficult but she growled impressively at any jock who tried to cross her.

Now Evelyn Capaldi is strolling around the edge of the tent and she's coming this way and I can hear her trilling, *"I need a drrrriiiink!"* with sort of a mock operatic flourish and when she sees me she pauses.

"You!" she chimes. "Hello, you!" She gives me a hug. She smells very good.

After she's gone off with her drink I ask Leigh, "She wouldn't remember my name, would she?" Not that I expected her to.

"Oh, in Evelyn's world, it doesn't matter," says Leigh.

"So you're Peter?" I ask Peter.

"Yep," Peter says.

"So, you get to wear a kilt." As long as we're being obvious here.

"Oh yeah. I like the kilt," he says. He's wearing some kind of traditional formal jacket, too, with epaulets and cords and double-breasted buttons. People always go on and on about how utterly *hot* guys in kilts are, but I find that chatting up a guy in a kilt feels more like an educational experience than a sexy one. It seems very Historical Village. I get the sense that I'm supposed to ask questions. I don't want to ask him whether he feels a breeze, and I really don't want to ask him that *other question* people always ask guys in kilts. So I say, "Are you getting a lot of weird questions about your kilt?"

"Like what?" he says.

"Oh, well—I don't know."

"I guess not," he says.

Then we stand watching the DJ set up his equipment for a while.

As Evelyn Capaldi makes her way through the tables to the dance floor she stops and puts her hand on Nicholas's arm. "When they play 'It's Raining Men' I *have* to get you boys out on the floor!"

"*No,*" Nicholas mouths across the table to me at the first opportunity. When she's out of earshot he says, "We are not doing the mandatory fabulous dance."

"Don't make us go out there," says Richard.

"I won't," I vow.

Peter, Round 2:

"Okay, I *do* have a question, actually," I tell him.

"Sure," he says.

"Okay, so the kilt is cool and all, but what if you got to dress up as, like, a *pirate* for a wedding party, would you?" Personally and even when I'm sober I think this is a great idea.

"A pirate?"

"You know, wear a puffy shirt? And a patch and stuff?"

"Why would I want to do that?" he says.

Richard takes Mrs. Kendall out on the floor and I dance with some of Kelly's friends. Then I sit and watch people dancing. I look at the women; I pick out the thin women and look at their bare arms and at their legs in stockings. I stretch my own legs and cross them and I realize I'm studying them to see if they could pass; if I could stand next to everyone else. I think about what Richard said to me back at the hotel. Maybe I do want to be a line. I don't want to be noticed so much as I want to be part of the order of things.

"Are we having fun?" Leigh asks me. Of course, I tell her. She sits down in the chair next to me.

"And are we drunk yet?" she asks. Oh, yes. Well, almost.

"You look a little sad," she says. "But you look really good, too."

My rose from the bouquet toss is on the table. Instead of doing a traditional bouquet toss, Kelly took a tip from *Martha Stewart Weddings* and threw a bunch of long-stemmed roses on the floor and all the single women scrambled to pick them up. Each rose has a fortune attached to it. Mine says, "After pain comes joy." If it looks like I am sad, I suppose that's why: I'm waiting.

"I tried talking to that Peter guy," I say. He is over across the tent talking with Evelyn Capaldi. Her dress is very retro garden party, pale pink with big peonies. It's the kind of dress I never felt I could pull off. To be honest, I don't think she can pull it off either.

"How did that go?" Leigh asks.

"Eh," I say.

Evelyn seems to be having much better luck. Peter is letting her poke him with her rose, which she also uses to sort of bawdily play with the hem of his kilt. Evelyn Capaldi, I have to admit, sort of has it going on; I bet her rose says something good.

I show Leigh the rose fortune. "Joy, huh?" she says. "It'll be about time."

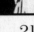

in the third person

Whenever someone clicks over to my site from somewhere else, the address of the place where it came from is recorded in a log, a long list of websites that I can't stop poring over. I keep clicking on each one to look. Most of them are online journals or weblogs; most of them are by women or girls. Their sites go by all kinds of titles, like *Rants and Ravens* or *Another Day* or *SubwayGrrl* or *Kitten Whip* or even just *Marla's Journal*; they'll have tagline descriptions like *Random Thoughts of a Twentynothing* or *My Myriad Misadventures* or *Nonstop Bitchfest*.

Sometimes *Pound* is just included in their lists of "Favorite sites," other times they'll mention something I wrote, or my site, or me. I saw the sentence "Today *Pound* had a funny story about Weight Watchers," on one site, and it took me a moment to recognize myself as *Pound*; it sounded oracular and weird. Once or twice I've been called

Wendy of Pound, which sounds pretty dorky, like I'm a *Star Wars* character or something. However, for most of the other sites I'm just *Wendy*, like I'm a Wendy they know. "I was thinking about what Wendy said the other day," someone I've never met will write. It gives me a prickly amnesiac sensation. I said what? When?

Clicking through the referral log is a lot like overhearing a few dozen conversations at once, all of them cued up to the moment where my name comes up. But then it's more than listening in; it's like peering through the skylight into a strange room. People have husbands or boyfriends with nicknames (Captain, TBone, Mr. Marla); they go on job searches; watch *Buffy*; paint their bedrooms; see movies that I've been meaning to get to; complain about their cars; fight with their mothers; mention other sites, including mine, in passing. When I visit these sites, I feel a little like a ghost who's been summoned by accident and then lingers. For almost a week I followed one girl's account of being home sick with the flu and watching nothing but *Real World* marathons. Every day, she claimed, a different cast member would make her throw up.

Elsewhere, someone named Jenna is recovering from a spectacular breakup in Colorado. There's a woman in Seattle whose name I don't know—I just know her page has a big photo of dewy roses on it; she's just joined a gym.

They're not all far away, these women, and I find I pay a little more attention to the sites of the ones who live in Chicago. I become familiar with Lexy, who takes classes at Columbia College and often goes to concerts I wish I'd known about before. She wrote me a fan email once. "You fucking rock so hard," she'd said. Sometimes she goes to Big Chicks—or so I read—and she'll complain about how oddly touchy-feely some of the gay guys are just because she's fat. I look through her site to find her picture so I'll know her if we're ever in the same place.

A couple weeks later a girl named Sarah writes me. "My friend Lexy turned me on to your site," she says, and when she says she has a site, too, I already know who she is: Likes Indian food, works on the same block I used to work downtown, has a boyfriend named Josh. Lexy linked to her and then she linked to me.

None of this feels as strange as I suppose it must be. It feels like it's the same old systems of chance and coincidence and proximity at work, the same imaginary diagram lines between everyone—people you know, people you haven't met yet, the ones you may have encountered according to some law of probability. Only now it feels like someone flipped a switch; now, the whole map is lit up and suddenly I can see my way to someone else.

I write her back. I know supposedly when you have fans *they're* supposed to stalk you, but whatever.

#

why oh why can't i

Tonight on TV there is a movie about the life of Judy Garland: *Me and My Shadows*. It stars Judy Davis as Judy, with some younger actress playing Teen Judy. I have been watching from the beginning and I almost believe all the Judys are one person; a Judy for real.

The studio tells her she's too fat and she believes it. You can see that she believes it. Or that she doesn't want to believe it but she has to. In one scene she walks through the studio lot looking at people looking at her.

I can't remember seeing Judy Garland in anything besides *The Wizard of Oz*, though I know I must have.

Judy Garland can't eat because the studio tells her so. She tells Mickey Rooney, "Gosh, I sure wish I could just have a hot dog." In the next scene she takes some pills.

Then Judy Garland's on speed, and she takes pills and she stumbles and her pills scatter everywhere and then she picks them up and pops them in her mouth. I kind of live for the pill-spilling scenes in movies like this. This is how you know things are getting bad. I get a bowl of cereal but I have to keep watching.

When I was a kid I always forgot the beginning of *The Wizard of Oz* was in black and white. It aired on TV only once a year and every year for a while I was convinced there was a mistake—something wrong with my memory or the TV station or the universe. It was hard to sit through the tornado scene and wait until Dorothy's house fell still. It would come as a relief when she got up and opened the door and made everything change.

Judy Garland is craving sundaes and chocolate cake and it strikes me how good these things sound, even as she's popping pills and falling into crumpled heaps and getting up and popping more pills. I get up for more cereal but I wish I had something better, because I would like to eat for Judy.

to want me

All afternoon one day I keep clicking on the email with the subject line *RSVP Lisa's Karaoke Bday Thursday 6/29*. I'm sure I know a Lisa but I don't know how. Eventually I figure it out: she's Lexy. I knew Lexy was a nickname but I didn't know what for, and now she's put me on her group email list. I'm supposed to reply with a Yes or No or Maybe, and I go with *maybe*, though already I have this idea that I'll show up.

I have the idea all week; until Thursday evening when I happen to put on a shirt that I bought recently to celebrate (and emphasize) taking off another five pounds, and think why the hell not, I'll go. I feel enough like the Wendy of my website to be seen in person. I feel good enough to take the el instead of driving, and I look at myself in the windows and imagine that I'm being wondered about.

The karaoke bar is in sort of an out-of-the-way neighborhood, and it's a weeknight, so it's not crowded; when I go walk in I see there's only one group—a dozen or so people taking up a few cocktail tables. They're very appreciatively watching someone up on the plywood stage platform, and I look over and see that it's Lexy all right. She's singing "Born to Be My Baby" by Bon Jovi.

Lexy is a lot bigger than me. I knew this because she said so, but a little part of me goes, *Wow, she's a big girl.* She is wearing all black but she's showing some cleavage; she's got on some kind of vintage hat—a little cloche with a mesh veil—and she's wearing a necklace with rhinestone letters that spell out BITCH. She's so much more of a spectacle than I could ever hope to be. She's belting out the Miss Ross and I'm standing near the door watching her, and I don't want to walk across the room; the place is big and even with her party it's a long empty way and everyone will see me, and either nobody knows me or everybody knows me. Oh, and there's the bar.

There are more songs and people I don't know are getting up and singing them. Every now and then there is a break between songs and as soon as I get the chance I say hi to Lexy, who hugs me. "I'm drunk," she says.

"I'm glad," I tell her.

She leads me over to one of the tables. "This girl! She has the website! The one I'm always talking about!" People nod. "Was I telling you about her website?" Not quite as much nodding. I sit down next to a girl who says, "So, you have a website?" Yes, I tell her. "How did you do that?" she asks.

"Uh, put my site online?" I ask.

"Right. I mean, was it hard?" She's being very nice about trying to give a shit.

"Oh, no. Not at all."

I get another drink. More people are coming in now: other groups filling in the tables around us (karaoke tends to be a tribal activity; you travel with your peeps, your K-posse, whatever), or else joining our party. Lexy's friend Sarah is here now. I recognize her from her bangs. She wrote a journal entry on her site about how she cut them too short; she'd put up a photo of just her forehead and yet, go figure, I recognize her from that.

"Hey, so I'm Wendy," I tell her.

"So you know Lisa?" she says. She seems to be watching one of the video monitors behind me.

"Yeah, well, I guess *you* know her more than I do, since you're friends and all," I'm saying, "and I just met her tonight, like, in person, and now I'm meeting you." In the middle of all this I realize she has no idea what I'm talking about. "You know, we've emailed . . . and stuff. You're *Sarah*, right? *The Mistress* Sarah?" I don't know why it sounds so wrong to say someone's Internet nickname out loud, but it does.

"Oh!" she says, looking straight at me. "Are you *Wendy* Wendy?"

I guess I am.

"I Want You to Want Me" by Cheap Trick is really an excellent karaoke selection because two-thirds of the song is nothing but WANT and NEED and LOVE and BEG.

Anyone can nail that part; the human id doesn't make mistakes. There are other lyrics to the song but seeing as how they are totally incomprehensible in the original recordings (especially the *Live at the Budokan* version), you are not obligated to do more than mumble those parts.

> Example:
> Didn't I, didn't I, didn't I see you cryin'?
> Oh, didn't I, didn't I, didn't I see you cryin'?
> *Feelalalawithouwafrenlalalafeela* dyin'?!

Really, don't even *look* at the lyrics monitor. You may wish to add occasional stage proclamations such as HELLO JAPAN!!!! so as to better simulate the arena rock experience. It goes without saying you need to be drunk for this.

"I heart you," says Sarah. Sarah sings "Summer Nights" from *Grease* with her friend James and I heart *her*.

Over at the next table someone has brought Lexy a present wrapped in pages of full-color hardcore porn and she screams with laughter.

There is a two-man duet of "I Got You Babe." Some guy sings "Lola" and we all sing along. Lexy is mostly busy drinking birthday shots and going back up to the stage for repeat performances, but Sarah and I have been hitting it off. She lets me smoke some of her cigarettes.

"At first I didn't even tell my boyfriend I was doing Weight Watchers," she says, handing me a cigarette. "Like it's such an Oprah thing to do. But then I had to bitch to someone about the meetings. They're retarded." We compare Weight Watchers drinking techniques ("Stoli Vanil and diet orange soda? Way better than it sounds," says Sarah), talk about online personals (it's how she met Josh), and discuss one of the scraps of the porno wrapping paper that are being passed around the group.

"Do you ever get in one of those moods where you just want to bend down and grab your ankles with joy?"

"I like her come-hither look."

"*Her* hither is very clean-shaven."

She lets me have another cigarette. It's getting late and the two guys she came in with, James and some tall guy with glasses, come by our table to say they're leaving. Sarah and I have just gotten another round so we're staying, she tells them.

James nods and says good-bye. The tall guy with the glasses says, "Bye. Nice to not even meet you or anything."

"Uh, okay, bye," I say, because he seems to be talking to me for some reason.

"That was my roommate Nathan," Sarah says after they've left. "Remember I pointed him out when he was singing 'Lola'?"

"Maybe you did." But I was watching the video. I wasn't paying attention.

"I wonder what was up with *him*," says Sarah.

rosy perfection

The fall/winter mandatory chore at my parents' house was going through my grandmother's photo collection; the spring/summer chore is to clean out the basement for their garage sale. My brother and I are getting dinner out of the deal, plus we can bring our own stuff to sell.

Part of the basement is my dad's office, and he turns up his stereo so we can all listen to Wagner as we go through the junk. The music lends a sense of dramatic discovery to pretty much every piece of crap we come across, though there's not all that much besides dusty, tangled bunches of old plastic flowers, grocery sacks, old paperbacks, and yet another stash of unused photo albums that my grandmother bought a couple years ago.

I open a box that contains pieces from what I think is a coffee percolator, a big wrinkled envelope full of recipe clippings and then, a stash of recipe cards in a beige plastic case with a clear lid. The box and the cards are starting to turn yellow, and on the bottom of each card on the recipe side it says *Copyright Weight Watchers 1974*.

"Where did you get these?" I ask my mom.

"I don't remember. I think we sent away for them," she says.

I flip through the cards. The color saturation in the photos is a little off, and some of the less timeless kitchenware trends of the '70s are represented alongside the food. There are a number of perfectly good recipes like chicken cacciatore and gazpacho, and then there are things like "Frankfurter Spectacular," which, as far as I can tell, is an upright pineapple encased in hot dogs—hot dogs split lengthwise and attached with toothpicks to form a terrifying fist of pork.

"What the hell?" I say, turning over the card. "These are Weight Watchers? There's no calorie information."

"They didn't do it that way back then," my mom says. "You had to just follow the program really closely. You had to make your own ketchup."

"Ugh, seriously?" A couple of older women who read my site have written me to tell me about how Weight Watchers used to be; how you had to make tuna salad with mustard instead of mayonnaise, eat liver once a week, and not have any snacks except for wet cigarette butts, so I guess I had some idea, but still.

"You're lucky, my dear," Mom says.

I can't stop flipping through the cards. I come across one for "Rosy Perfection Salad": shredded red cabbage in an aspic mold. Just a big, wet bale of red cabbage. I look at

it more closely and see that it's served with a garnish of . . .
shredded red cabbage.

"What are you laughing so hard at?" my mom asks.

"Can I have these?" I beg her.

"What for, to cook with them?"

"I don't know," I tell her. "Just to look at, I guess."

I've brought a load of my old fat clothes—a suitcase, two
plastic bags, and then a shopping bag full, all stuffed into
the backseat of my car. I kept a lot of old things packed
away in my storage stall in the basement of my building,
as if I'd been stockpiling for some kind of fashion apoca-
lypse. I seem to have created some kind of clothing land-
fill with distinct strata, and at the very bottom I found
baffling things from 1995: long tunic tops and big,
smocky Lane Bryant sweater vests. I can't tell if I was
really that heavy, or if that's just the style I preferred, or
if that was the kind of stuff everyone else was wearing
back then.

"I remember when you got that," my mom says when I
hold up a pinafore dress. I got it for my first real job after
college: an assistant job at a textbook company. A fucking
pinafore, from JCPenney, with businesslike black and
brown stripes over a white blouse with a shawl collar.

"I can't believe I thought this was me," I tell my mom.
I remember I didn't really like it, but sometimes I almost
enjoyed the austerity. I would wear it and pretend I was
Stout Clara, the Dumpiest Brontë Sister of Them All.
Weekday mornings I'd trudge up to the el platform and
stand in the wind and think of the moors.

I don't remember if I was happy back then. I suppose I could have been, but I can't tell from the clothes.

After dinner I ask my dad if he can take some photos of me with his new digital camera. "I just want to see if I can tell how much weight I've lost," I explain.

I don't tell him that I wanted to put them on my website and that an average of hundred and seventy-one people a day (according to my site stats) are going to look at them.

I stand in the living room of my parents house trying to act normal; to be just ever so casually caught in the act of being twenty-five pounds lighter.

My dad takes four pictures while my mom calls out advice.

"Just put your arms down," she says, since instinctively I am holding them the way I hold them in the mirror; sort of floating out my side like an interpretive dancer. I try them bent akimbo with my hands on my hips. I would like to show some personality, after all. "Don't worry about that," my mom calls out. "They're just progress pictures, right?"

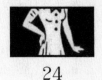

little man

I have at least twenty black shirts, all in different sizes and in various permutations of sleeve lengths and necklines and shades of black. I keep buying more black shirts, too; new black shirts that fit me better than the old black shirts. Sometimes I think I need a special infrared light in my closet so I can find everything.

Today I am trying things on. I am weeding out things that have gotten too big, and finding smaller things that I can fit into again. The black T-shirt I've just pulled over my head doesn't fit too tightly and the sleeves hit in just the right place. I tug at the hem and stick my chest out. I like this shirt; when did I buy it? I have no idea. The tag inside says it's a Gap basic T-shirt, size medium. And then I realize it's not my shirt at all: it's Stuart's.

*   *   *

Stuart was only an inch or two shorter than I am, which makes him short for a guy, not freakishly short; but his build was somewhat slight. Next to a tall, plump girl like me, he was damn near petite.

The night he first hit on me I'd gone out dancing with Leigh; she'd brought along some of her regulars, including Stuart. I remember at some point I was out on the dance floor and looked down to find him sort of caught in my cleavage like a piece of Kleenex. *Well, hello there, little man!* I thought. He came with all sorts of darling accessories like a cell phone and a laptop and teeny wire-rimmed glasses.

I found the whole situation hilarious at times, though sometimes I felt a little uncomfortable next to him—outsized, like the Sensational She-Hulk.

One night I pointed out that he usually dated women who were more his size. "Is it weird for you that I'm different?" I asked him. Stuart had advanced degrees in linguistics and more books than anyone else I had ever dated. He made a point of being the smartest person in the room, though more often than not the room was a bar. Still he was bright and I wanted to know what kind of answer he'd come up with.

"Well, I think there are definite evolutionary preferences for big healthy women to perpetuate the species," he'd said. "As opposed to skinny little Victoria's Secret models."

I wanted to like his answer. I also wanted to say *Yeah, whatever; now climb up on Momma's lap because you know you want it, you damn Cub Scout.* But I didn't.

Stuart was twice divorced and he had a photo of Laeticia Casta on his computer's desktop. Once I heard him say "Hello, Laetica!" out loud to it as he booted up the machine. He was forty-two and didn't have children. I don't know what evolutionary preference that reflected. He did seem to have a knack for perpetuating himself as a bad memory.

Psychologically, being wronged by Stuart was like that final segment in *Trilogy of Terror* where that little doll torments Karen Black and stabs her with his itty-bitty spear and bites her. I mean it was that freaky and humiliating. "I don't get why you didn't just kick his ass or really tell him off," Richard says sometimes. *You think I didn't try?* I want to tell him. *You think Karen Black wasn't trying when she shoved that Zuni doll in the oven?*

A couple months after we'd broken up I saw him at Shucker's. He was relentlessly jolly as he tried to talk to me from a few bar stools away. "How goes the world of children's publishing?" he called out. "Shut up, little man," I said, just loud enough for Leigh to hear me as she tended the bar.

He'd left the T-shirt along with a pair of boxer shorts in a green paisley pattern. I used to hold up the boxers and grimly consider how small they were. I showed them to Richard once. "I guess I should throw these out," I said.

"No, keep them," Richard had said. "Think of them as Lucky Leprechaun Pants. You can put them on a keychain." I tossed them anyway.

But I'd forgotten about the shirt. I'd come across it once before when I'd put it with some stuff to donate to the Salvation Army, but at some point after that my closet got disorganized again, and the shirt wound up at the bottom of my closet where I picked it up and put it on.

In all the diet or makeover stories I've read it's supposed to be a big moment when the heroine can fit into her old homecoming dress, or a pair of size six jeans, or a white two-piece bathing suit—something in which they become the thin person they once were or else always very wistfully dreamed of being. I wonder what I'm meant to get from standing here in Stuart's shirt.

I don't think I've changed at all. The shirt smells slightly of Chanel Egoiste, which still makes me shudder the way it always did. What's different now is that Stuart the Little Man isn't all that little. The thing that made him specific to me suddenly isn't true anymore. Now Stuart could be anyone. I suppose I can be anyone, too.

#

wish upon

Once you were fat, and maybe now you're still fat, technically speaking, but let's say *once upon a time* you were fat for
the purposes of the story. In fairy tales you're only really
different once—you might change and change back if the
spell is tough, but eventually time stops moving forward
and the ever after kicks in.

Once upon a time you were fat and you lived in your fat
like a castle. Now, so the story goes, it's a glass casket, and
some guy will come along and see you in it. If you're lucky,
he'll fall for you either despite it or because of it. You'd love
to know which one for sure but you're supposed to stay
dead until it happens; you don't get to wake up until he's
there.

steps

Sarah writes to tell me she had fun meeting me the other night. "Incidentally, my roommate told me he thinks you're pretty," she says. "Do with that information what you will." I am trying to remember his name and his face. I can just remember glasses but I can't tell you what kind, even.

I am putting new photos up on the website, the ones my dad took of me last month. I seem to be squinting in most of them. I look at them hard to try and figure out what it is about them that keeps me from looking the way I do in the mirror. Something about the colors in the picture and the objects around me: I am a girl in a purple shirt standing in some house somewhere and you can't tell anything has transpired. The pictures are incidental and still, and, on their own, they don't look like progress at all.

They do look different next to the karaoke pictures. They show that I am smaller than the flailing woman in the glitter sunglasses, and—in more ways than one—more contained.

I use Adobe Photoshop to change the pictures to black and white to match the older pictures. And then my instinct is to hide my eyes, because they're covered in the earlier photos, too.

I click on the zoom controls and enlarge the image and scroll up to the part of the photo where my face is. I was smiling too hard and my eyes are pinched, so I guess it's partly out of vanity that I'm hiding them now. With a few clicks and a drag of the mouse I've drawn a little box around my eyes. Then I fill in the box with black. I do the same thing with the second photo. When I'm done it doesn't look so much like me posing awkwardly for a web page anymore. With the bars over my eyes it looks like my life is elsewhere.

When I put the photos up I get emails from a handful of people who tell me I need to put up more pictures. One reader says she wants to "follow every step."

I go to my Weight Watchers meetings, every week, and they write down my weight on a card and I put the card in my bag and go home and then, these days, most of my effort goes into doing the exact same thing I did the week before, and if the week before wasn't the best week, I try to faithfully reenact another week where I lost a pound. All it feels like I'm doing is repeating the same experiment every week with all the same basic elements: Kashi cereal, and Monday-Wednesday-Friday gym, and veggie burgers for lunch. Sometimes it feels like I'm winding myself around something, like I'm going in circles that get tighter with each lap; that my lead gets shorter with each step. So I think I hate *steps*. I would rather just run and not look back until the distance is unmistakable.

The same woman also wrote in her email to me, "You are an inspiration."

I still don't want to look back.

More emails:

> *Why did you put bars over your eyes? Nathan (my roommate) was kind of disappointed. Let's hang out again soon.*
>
> XO, Sarah

> hi,
> *i'm sure you get a lot of these, but i just wanted to say that i'm really glad your website exists. It makes me laugh about things i didn't think i could laugh about, things i actually want to cry about. i'm so grateful for that. i know you keep this journal for you, or at least primarily for you, but i just wanted to tell you—whether it means anything to you or not—that i'm just really glad i found it.*
>
> best, Krista

> *Dear Wendy,*
> *I'm writing on behalf of the JournalCon committee to invite you to come speak in October. As you may know, JournalCon Chicago is the second annual gathering of on-*

line journallers, diarists, and webloggers from all around the country. We are tentatively planning a panel about weight loss journals and body image and we would be extremely honored to have you as a speaker. If you're interested we hope you'll respond as soon as possible. We look forward to hearing from you! Sincerely, Jessamyn

I am on the elliptical trainer thinking *I am someone's inspiration.* I think I ought to be motivated by the idea that I am someone's inspiration. I am walking without making steps, which is the whole point of the elliptical trainer.

Every step is a glide; every step is suspended. I feel like I'm making my way with puppet feet, which is not exactly inspirational, but maybe there's something in the way I push and push and pedal this thing.

I grew up a good swimmer and I could tread water in the deepest area of the park district pool. Sometimes when I did, it wasn't enough that I could hold myself up—I would see how steady I could be; I tried to limit all movement to just the treading, the necessary motion, my arms working; my feet efficiently churning the colder water from the bottom. I could do it for only so long before I'd pitch over to the side. Now on the trainer I think I remember the motion I was trying to sustain, though it's not quite the same thing.

26

0. anonymous

I was fourteen and doing my mom a favor: I sat at the dining room table copying a logo and the words *Overeaters Anonymous* onto a sheet of typing paper.

My mom had given me one of her books, where the OA logo appeared on the back cover. I had to make it big enough for a sign; a sign that my mom would put up on the bulletin board of our church to advertise the Tuesday evening meetings for Overeaters Anonymous. I couldn't just trace it but I didn't believe in tracing things anyway. I could draw and I was going to use my eyes.

It didn't take me very long to draw the logo itself: it was blocky and stylized and looked like it was for a very dull company. I struggled more over the letters of the accompanying words. The A was tilted in a way that I knew was supposed to be artful but to me it looked awkward.

I understood what Alcoholics Anonymous was. My

mother was a substance abuse counselor and her job was to help people get through the Twelve Steps, starting with Admit You Have a Problem. I knew from television movies that *Not* Admitting You Have a Problem invariably meant you had one and you had it bad. It meant that you had a bathtub full of empty bottles and maybe you fell down spectacularly in public. It seemed to be an especially showy kind of ruin, much better than just being fat.

As abbreviations went, AA had an obvious symmetry, but OA sounded awful to my ears; the O was conspicuous and seemed to call attention to itself, which was the last thing that fat people needed, I thought.

I don't know how it got started with my mom and me and the ice cream. Ice cream was one of the few things my mother could keep down in the years after her stomach stapling surgery.

Certain foods got "stuck"—bread, some kinds of meat, solid things. When she'd first gotten the surgery she could only have liquids and stuff in puree form. There was baby food in the refrigerator and it was hers. Two weeks after her first surgery she'd craved meat. She'd taken a cooked hamburger and tried to mash it up as much as humanly possible, even putting it in the blender for a few seconds. She couldn't keep it down and got sick on the kitchen floor. I was eleven and had never seen my mother throw up before. She'd always taken care of me when I had stomach flu, which made it even more uncomfortable to watch her clean up after herself.

Ice cream, however, went down without much trouble;

she discovered this right away. So she ate ice cream, and she'd have a lot of it.

I was becoming intimately familiar with the insides of half-gallon ice cream boxes. Ice cream has a life of its own inside a box like this. It has an elaborate, though short, history that begins with the layer made smooth and even by the lid of the box—the part that goes soft first, that is maybe at its very best consistency when it is first brought home from the store. We'd still all be putting groceries away when I'd take out the ice cream. My mom would see what I was doing and get the bowls out for us.

After a few servings, the thing to do was dig out the middle and leave the rest of the ice cream packed against the sides of the box. The sides were the best, supple against the spoon and yielding just enough to scoop out a little here and there, straight out of the box. Or else one could sit down with the box and simply steal and steal and steal. It was stealing because each bite had nothing to do with the next one or the last.

I usually went for the flavors with ripples and stripes because they made for purposeful excavation. And I liked Neopolitan, with its orderly three-flavor rigor. It appealed to me also because of its name: compared to all the other flavors of ice cream *Neopolitan* sounded fancy and abstract. I would sit down at the kitchen table with an open carton and explore various Neopolitan propositions: was the divide between chocolate and strawberry an arbitrary line, or was it a plane? Was it perfectly parallel to the vanilla/strawberry divide? I'd inquire with my spoon.

We usually bought the brands in boxes that opened at

the short end; the ones that had the flap that said "Please Fold This Side In First," and I liked entertaining the idea that I might close the box again sometime.

My mom was getting fat again. The surgeries could only do so much; unlike the kinds of gastric surgeries that came later, there was no intestinal bypass; all the doctors had done was create a smaller stomach pouch, and it was possible to stretch the stomach over time.

When I was in junior high she started going to OA.

"The whole idea is that you can be addicted to food," she explained.

There was a part of me that found this concept hilarious. I imagined a clichéd AA meeting with hazy rooms and shaky, pale, ex-barflies swigging coffee and chain-smoking and confessing in hoarse but steady voices. I pictured them all with thought balloons over their heads showing pretty cakes, and glistening turkeys, and gooey Snickers bars being very professionally pulled apart, like on the commercials.

"Well, it's not *quite* like that," my mom said. "But, well, sort of."

It seemed inscrutably sad to have to think about food like that.

Ice cream, I decided, was for another kind of thinking, an opposite kind: when I went to eat it I already had my thoughts in place.

I thought my mom shouldn't be eating so much damn ice cream, and I thought I'd better do something before she got to it and finished the whole thing—often she would, the same night it was bought. Then somebody would buy more because there had to be more. I hated this need for more, and so I ate as much of the ice cream as I could as soon as I could. I did it to defeat need, I thought. My mom said she was powerless over food and I thought it was the stupidest fucking thing I'd ever heard in my life.

The fridge was just to the left of the kitchen doorway. I could open the freezer door and grab the ice cream while my mom sat at the table with her back to me. Sometimes she was talking on the phone—sometimes, with her OA sponsor—and the phone cord was stretched across the doors of the refrigerator. I'd hold the cord just so, so that my mom wouldn't feel the pull or the slack; I'd take the box out of the freezer and close the door softly. I'd eat it in another room with the spoon I'd saved.

I always counted on her not to notice.

good company

"Nathan will be a little late. He insisted on riding his bike up here," says Sarah. "He told us to go ahead and rent his shoes and make sure they have his size. God." She hauls out a pair of red and blue bowling shoes and puts them on the table. They're so big it's like he's already there.

I'm with Sarah and her boyfriend, Josh, at Waveland Bowl waiting for a lane to open up.

"This is the girl with the website," she tells Josh.

"You have a website, too, honey," says Josh.

"Yeah, but that's different," says Sarah. "Wendy's sort of famous."

I am working on an expression to wear whenever someone says something like this. I sort of roll my eyes a little and then shake my head shyly. "No," I say. "It's just because I write for that Television Without Pity site. They get a lot of traffic." I concentrate on playing with Nathan's shoes on the table. I crash them together like two stunt cars. I will be meeting him soon.

After the third or fourth time Sarah mentioned Nathan to me in her emails I had to write her back and confess that I couldn't remember what he looked like. She replied right away and attached a photo of a guy with hipster geek glasses and a sort of solemn expression. The photo would only display sideways ("Sorry, I don't know how to fix it," wrote Sarah) so I had to sort of tilt my head to look at it properly. In the photo, Nathan was holding up a bicycle. I studied the building behind him; it looked like it might be in Wicker Park. I could see a couple of little tattoos on his bicep. I hoped he was as tall as I remembered him.

I wrote back and thanked Sarah for sending the picture. "Does this mean he wants to meet me or something?" I wrote.

"Does this mean you want to meet him, too?" she wrote back.

Nathan is late but when he does show up he's tall. He has the biggest shoulders I've ever seen. Like I wonder how he gets them through the door.

"You're late," Sarah says,

"I had a flat," he says.

"A *flat?*" Sarah says exasperatedly.

"Flat like your ass," he says.

"*You're* an ass," Sarah shoots back.

Apparently, Nathan is an ex of Sarah's; she mentioned this earlier. Now they're like a cranky brother and sister, snapping each other's elastic, so to speak. Or at least I'll try to think of them as siblings. He keeps looking over to where I'm sitting.

I wave. "Hey, I'm Wendy," I say. "Again."

"I know," he says. "Nice of Sarah to introduce us."

"Shut up," says Sarah. "Wendy, this is Nathan Pelley." Nathan waves back.

"It's *not* flat," Josh says.

"What? Oh, thank you, sweetie," says Sarah. She goes back to tying her bowling shoes.

Nathan catches my eye to make sure I see him trying not to laugh.

We bowl only one game. The alley is full of families with kids playing Bumper Bowl and sometimes it's easier to be distracted by the sight of a four-year-old dropping a massive ball than it is to talk. Nathan does take the time to point out that the balls I bowl travel even slower than some of the children's efforts. It's true: all my balls seem to go about 16 rpm.

"It looks like it's going *backwards*," he says, when I try to take out a spare two pins. "I swear, the sun is going to flare out and die before your ball gets there."

I'm thinking Nathan is the kind of guy who, in junior high, would have stolen the Thompson Twins pin off my purse and sent it skidding across the classroom floor like a hockey puck. Maybe it's time I dealt with a guy like this. Back then, all I'd do was cry.

By the time we get to the bar I know that Nathan works as a manager at Barnes & Noble—"I mean, whatever, I get a lot of books," he says; he grew up in the west suburbs; he has about eight hundred CDs; he's obsessed with '60s British movies; and he reads anything he can find about Dutch Schultz.

After just one round of drinks Sarah says she and Josh are going to make it an early night. "Josh has kind of an upset stomach," she says. "I mean, if *you* guys want to stay out, don't let us stop you."

"You won't," says Nathan.

I'll take that as a sign I'm good company.

"That guy Josh is always about to puke or something," says Nathan after they leave. "I can't stand him."

The bar around us is starting to fill up. Nathan gets up to put money in the jukebox and he comes back with a pitcher of beer.

"So, you know, I have this website," I start to tell him.

"Yeah, Sarah won't shut up about it," Nathan says. "She's always all, like, 'Wendy said the funniest thing today! Wendy says that Pirate's Booty snacks are the best!' You're like her Oprah."

"Are you making fun of me?"

"No, I mean, I read your site," he says. "I think it's funny. Like that comic strip in the paper. What's it called? *Cathy?*"

Just for that, I'm taking one of his cigarettes.

"You get I'm kidding, right?" he says.

"Light my fucking cigarette," I tell him.

"So what are you going to write your next entry about?" he asks.

"I don't know. I was thinking maybe I'd write about that movie where Gwyneth Paltrow wears the fat suit."

"I have an idea," says Nathan. "Why don't you write about *chocolate*? Like how much you *love* it."

"Oh, yeah," I say. "Chocolate and *shopping*."

"*Shoe* shopping," he adds. "I bet you live for shit like that."

"Why don't they make a chocolate shoe? You know?"

"You'd like that. You could eat them when you got one of your nutty female-type chocolate cravings."

"And then suddenly I WOULDN'T HAVE SHOES so then I'd need to GO SHOE SHOPPING SOME MORE."

"Do you have 'The PMS' right now or something?" he asks, making air quotes with his fingers.

I make air quotes back at him. "If it weren't for '*these*' you'd be '*dead*,' you know."

"Okay," he says over another pitcher. "I know I'm giving you shit about your site and stuff. So you should probably see this." He takes out his wallet and pulls out his ID. Right away I can tell his picture is very different.

"Your hair is brown," I say, studying the picture. He has it bleached blond now. I also notice that his neck is thicker in the photo, his chin less defined. "You were heavier?" The license shows his height as 6'3" and his weight well over 300 lbs.

"Yeah. I lost eighty pounds this past year," he says. "I don't know if Sarah ever mentioned it. I just decided to really try, and that's how I really got into riding my bike. I mean, I'm glad I did it, but it was hard, and sometimes it sucked, and, well—I guess I don't have to explain this."

"Right."

I'm listening to everything he's saying, but also I'm thinking: *eighty pounds*. I know men lose weight more quickly than women so I wonder how eighty Guy Pounds converts to compare with what I've lost.

"So I just wanted to let you know you shouldn't feel weird about being, you know, Amazing Diet Girl, or whatever," he says.

"Thanks."

"Because I mean, you're not totally stupid about it."

A Creed song starts playing on the jukebox. Nice and pompous.

"You picked this song out, right?" I ask him.

"No. *God*, no." He looks around as if to make sure nobody heard me. "*No*. You're not serious, right?"

"No, I was kidding."

"Are you *sure*?" he says.

"Yes." Jeez.

"I hope you know I was joking about the chocolate thing," he says.

"Yes, I know." I am pouring the last of the beer from the pitcher and when I look up he is watching my face; he seems to be waiting for me to smile.

"So what should I write about?" I ask him. "Seriously."

"I think you should write about, I don't know, this guy you met."

"Oh, *him*."

"Yeah." Under the table his knee is pressed up against mine.

FLUFFY MACKEREL PUDDING

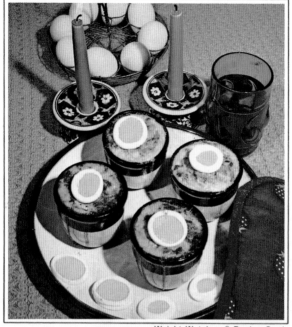

Weight Watchers® Recipe Cards

Once upon a time the world was young and the words *mackerel* and *pudding* existed far, far away from one another.

One day, that all changed. And then, whoever was responsible somehow thought the word *fluffy* would help.

Oh, and eggs, too.

SLENDER QUENCHERS

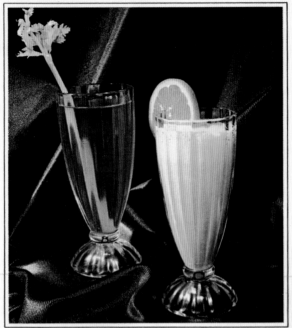

Weight Watchers® Recipe Cards

These are the saddest diet beverages ever.

The one on the right is skim milk and orange pulp. The one on the left is made with water, sherry extract, and two beef bouillon cubes.

No, really.

Well, there's also celery in it. Oh, and SELF-LOATHING.

CHILLED CELERY LOG

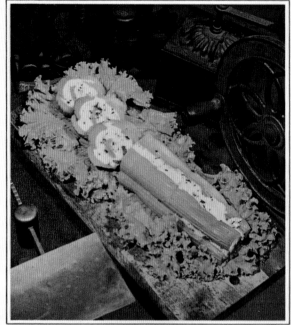

Weight Watchers® Recipe Cards

You could eat this log. Or, you could stick your hand in a rusty kitchen grinder. Yeah, have fun.

ONION SAUCE

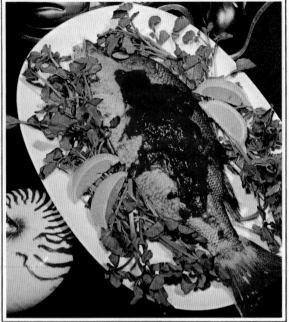

Weight Watchers® Recipe Cards

They call this "onion sauce" but it looks more like the end of a snuff film to me. *Fish* snuff. Die, fish, *die*.

INSPIRATION SOUP

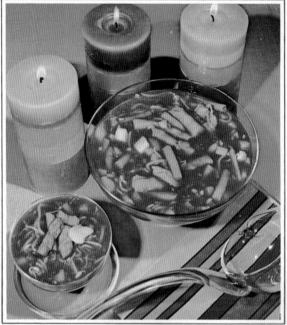

Weight Watchers® Recipe Cards

The Soup is Inspiration. The Soup is Love. Smell the Soup.

When one first arrives here, one may believe the Soup tastes *like ass*. That is not so, my child. The Soup is Inspiration and the Soup is Love. Your name is now "Harmonia." The Soup is Inspiration, and you do not want to leave. The Soup is Love, and we have an electrified fence. The Soup is Inspiration. And the Soup is Love.

MARCY'S "ENCHILADA"

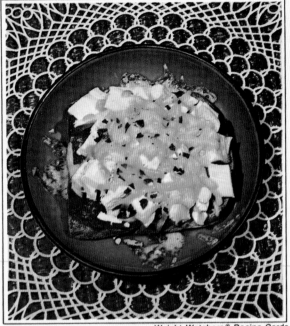

Weight Watchers® Recipe Cards

We don't know who "Marcy" is, only that she thinks "enchilada" is wacky Mexican talk for "shit on a shingle."

JELLIED TOMATO REFRESHER

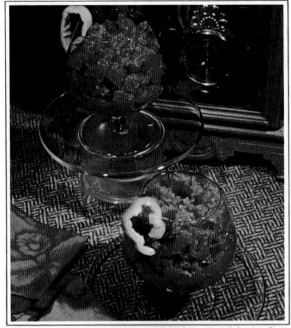

Weight Watchers® Recipe Cards

Yes, let's have these in *brandy snifters*. Let's just tip our heads back and let the chunks slide in.

The time you spent eating these is time you'll want back at the very end of your life. That's why they're served with a clock.

ROSY PERFECTION SALAD

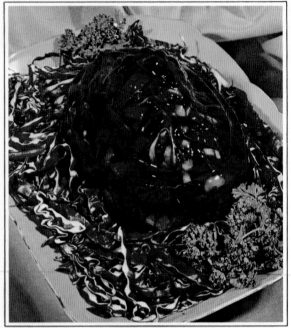

Weight Watchers® Recipe Cards

I don't think you're ready for this jelly.

I don't think you'll ever be. None of us will. No. No way.

FISH "TACOS"

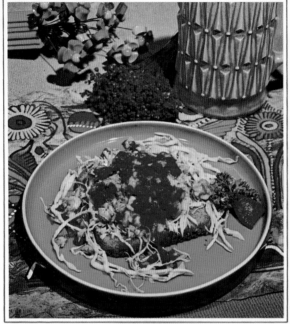

Weight Watchers® Recipe Cards

Mexican food is easy to make! All you need is toast and quotation marks! Just ask Marcy!

Marcy needs to be stopped.

I so do not understand the props here.

MOUSSE OF SALMON

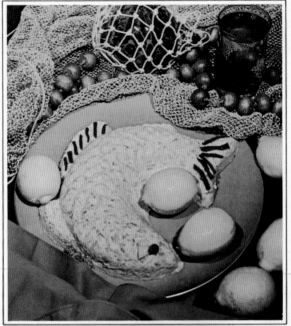

Weight Watchers® Recipe Cards

Sometimes salmon will come to the big city full of dreams. Only to wind up used, and mangled, and reconstituted, and all tarted up in some kind of sick, horrifying salmon drag.

Look, it's still trying to spawn. With lemons. It's confused. Oh, man, so sad.

FRANKFURTER PIE

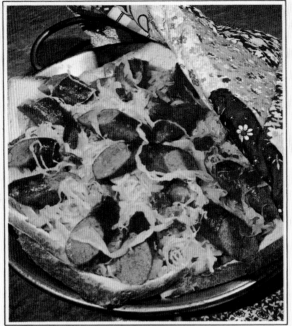

Weight Watchers® Recipe Cards

Frankfurters in a pie under a quilt.

You know how when you were a kid and you walked in on your parents? When you repressed the memory it wound up looking like this. Good luck with therapy.

FROZEN CHEESE SALAD

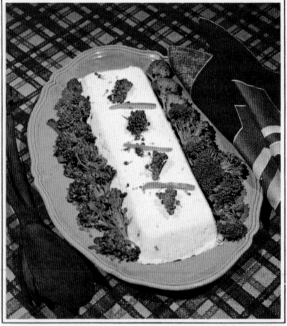

Weight Watchers® Recipe Cards

Well, *of course* it's a salad; there are wooden salad utensils next to it, see? You take the spoon and whack at the block of frozen cheese and…and…okay, nothing happens. Because it's *frozen cheese,* dumbass.

PARTY BURGERS

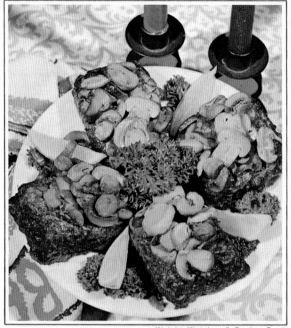

Weight Watchers® Recipe Cards

Woo! Party burgers! Burgers that *party*! Bunless burgers! Four-way naked burger action! Burgers gone WILD! Naked burgers, baby! See party burgers *totally garnish themselves and each other*! PARTY! Woo!

CRAB NEWBURG

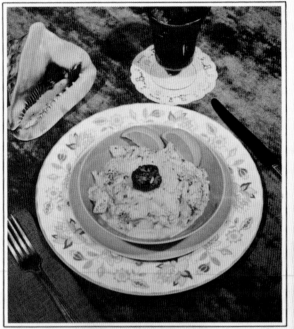

Weight Watchers® Recipe Cards

Wow, Crab Newburg on pink velvet, and it's only your first date with the Miami drug lord. And sweetie? He said it was white zinfandel but I wouldn't drink it too fast if I were you.

Hold the shell to your ear and you can hear heavy breathing, baby.

PEACHY CAKE

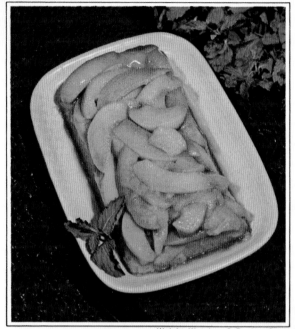

Weight Watchers® Recipe Cards

It was the '70s. Peaches already came in the requisite "goldenrod" color, but it took a little more work to make them modular enough for your space-age kitchen.

MOCK HERRING SALAD

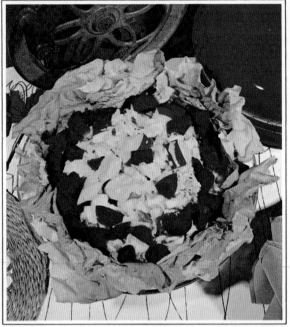

Weight Watchers® Recipe Cards

Mock Herring Salad all you want but it'll never cry. *You*, on the other hand, have to eat this shit.

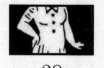

the nose thing

We're in my bed at eight o'clock on Monday night. It's dark out; when did it get dark?

We're kissing and sometimes we split a cigarette. The Marlboro Lights are his but I'm reaching for them more and more.

We talk when we smoke and when we don't smoke we're doing other stuff. I wonder when we'll get to a point where we're not either smoking or having sex. I wonder if Nathan is going to want to spend the night again.

I'm getting so used to his skin. I almost can't remember what it was like to look at him before I became familiar with his shoulder and the pink blotch on his upper arm and the way his chest hair is sparse enough to see each one, to see where it comes out of his skin. I know the landscape of his left side very well now. I'm actually a little tired of looking at the left arm with the Badz Maru tattoo on his bicep. He always takes this side of the bed and lies on his other arm.

"Why are you shifting around all of a sudden?" he says. I didn't think I was.

"I'm just getting some water," I tell him. "Want some?" I've been telling myself to *keep drinking water* as if I'm drunk, or running a marathon, or on a very long flight.

Nathan came over Friday night. It was our fourth date.

Saturday morning I dropped him off at his job at the bookstore; it was too far for him to ride from my apartment. I got out and waited on the sidewalk while he wrestled his bike out of the backseat of my car; he wouldn't let me help. When he finally got it free, he kept one hand lightly on the seat while he kissed me goodbye.

He told me to have a good day. I told him to have a good weekend, since it was Labor Day weekend, and people are always doing something.

"I'm not doing anything tonight," he said, "if you want to get dinner after I get off work."

"Oh. Oh, yeah. I could do that," I said. I wanted to get back in the car and whoop.

He looked over at his bike. "I guess I'll just, you know, lock this up."

Sunday morning I remembered I had to meet my friend Kristine for brunch at eleven.

"The front door just locks by itself," I told him.

"Cool," he mumbled, and turned over to go back to sleep.

He was sitting in the armchair flipping through a copy of *Bitch* magazine when I got back three hours later.

"Hey," he said. "I just have to put some pants on."

He did when we went to get dinner Sunday night at the Golden Angel Pancake House.

Monday we were there again for breakfast. Or something. It was almost two in the afternoon.

"Do you have to do anything today?" he asked. "It's a holiday, right?"

"Yeah. Everything's probably closed. All the stores and stuff." I looked out the window by our booth: it was sunny and warm. I tried to think of what people actually do in weather like this. Just walk around? "Let's take a nap when we get back."

"Good idea," Nathan said.

Sarah called Monday afternoon. "Is Nathan still there?" she asked. "He didn't come home last night and I figured he was with you, but . . ." She sounded a little concerned. "So he's still there, right?"

"Right. It's fine," I told her.

"Oh, my," she said.

I bring back water for both of us. Then, of course, I have to pee. "You keep running around," Nathan says.

In the bathroom I look myself over. I have a couple of odd bruises. I know one of them is from tripping on the pedal of his bicycle on my way to the kitchen. He'd brought it up to the apartment. "You should get one of those hooks to hang it on," he'd said. "Since you're in a studio and all."

I also have something vaguely hickeyish on my shoulder near my neck. Richard once told me that toothpaste gets rid of hickeys but I have no idea how it works. He also said a comb works, too; you run the teeth over your skin. I try it using Nathan's comb.

He has stuff in here; a shirt hanging up, a toiletries bag. I think he brought it Friday night. The comb hurts. I feel like I've got a bad sunburn all over. I'd feel raw if I didn't feel so overcooked at the same time.

"I have to go back to work tomorrow," I tell Nathan when I come out.

"You want me to stay?" he says.

"I don't want you to leave just yet," I say, and I hope he knows what I mean.

"Okay," he says. His hands are doing something. He's sort of tickling me. I have to tell him to stop.

"Sorry." Now he's just rubbing.

"Yeah, that's better," I tell him. It feels good but at the same time I want my skin back. It's been three days now.

"What are you doing?"

"Your nose is so cute," he says. He is pinching it gently. "I like your nose." He squeezes it tentatively and then wriggles the cartilage.

"Okay. Don't go sticking your fingers up there."

"Like *this*?"

"GOD!" I'm laughing, though. "Stop it!" "I just want to kiss your nose." He kisses it. Then he bites it a little.

"Hey . . ." I'm trying to turn my head to kiss him, to catch his mouth with mine. But he is not giving up the nose. He's sucking on it. Oh Jesus, that's enough. His wet teeth are grazing the sides.

"Uhh . . ." I say. Um, stop?

Then he clamps down hard. There's a horrifying suction, a sustained hydraulic slurping action. He's sucking my nose, he's doing it so hard I think it's going to dislocate. He needs to get off me because what if my nose pops and my sinuses implode and my eyeballs get dislodged and he doesn't even know, has no idea how much I hate this and how I might even die and everything.

I start screaming and when he pulls away my voice bursts out like I've been uncorked. *"Nnuuuuuuhh! Ayyyyaaaaaahhhh!"*

If it sounds like it comes from the feral depths of my being it's because *it is*. Because it's been *sucked out*.

"All right, all right," he says, a little panicked. I push him off me and I scoot back and catch my breath.

"Are you okay?" he says.

"I'm fine," I say. Then I start to cry uncontrollably. I curl up and put my hands to my face and bawl.

"Oh, shit," he says. *Oh shit* is right.

"I just wanted you to *stop*," I howl.

Really, I wanted him to stop everything and go home so I could look forward to the next time I saw him. But he wouldn't, and he stayed, and he molested my nose.

When I stop crying a little I get up out of bed and grab some sheets and stumble over to the bathroom. "Is my face all right? My nose?" I look in the mirror. It's purple. Sort of a purplish gray, and mottled just like a hickey. Nathan totally gave me a nose hickey.

When I come out he says, "Oh. Yeah. It's a little red."

I don't say anything and start grabbing up my clothes.

"I'm sorry," he says, bewildered. "I guess I'll go now." He is trying to laugh this off.

"Yeah, maybe you *should* go." I'm getting dressed. I think I'm serious. Like I ought to very seriously consider whether I want to pursue a relationship with a person like Nathan, a brutish nose-sucker with a poor sense of boundaries. Now I am picking up his clothes and putting them in a pile.

He gets up, too. "Fine, I'll go. I guess you need to think or something."

Elizabeth and I had discussed how there might be some physical anxieties about getting into a relationship again, body-image issues; I might be a little sensitive about certain parts of my body. Who the hell knew that my *nose* was one of them?

Nathan follows me around the apartment while I straighten things up. I'd made a little stack of books to lend him and now I make a point of picking a couple of them up. "I don't have to take those," he says.

"No. Here." I hand him the books. "Let's just talk tomorrow."

"First you have to tell me if we're going to do this again," he says. "Because I think you already know."

"You almost sucked my nose off my head."

"I know."

"So we're not going to do that again."

"What about everything else?"

"Probably."

"Good." He pulls me in to hug me and I let him.

He leaves the bike in the kitchen and I give him a ride home.

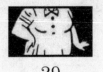

meter and magnet

Every day I visit my site statistics page to see my daily average of visits. Every day it changes. It's higher on Friday than it is on Monday because not as many people read me on the weekends. When I first started checking the statistics page I was getting just under a hundred visitors a day. Now I am up to around two hundred and fifty.

I can see a graph that shows me how many visitors are in each time zone all over the world. Most of the visitors are in Eastern Standard Time. I guess that's probably because there is a higher population density. I try not to think about how more people understand me there than in my own time zone, Central Standard.

Sometimes the bar graph will show a little stump in one of the time zones below Australia, and every now and then it shows a little sliver in the time zone that contains China. I wonder how many of these hits are accidents. I wonder if there is anything I say on my site that makes a difference. I know the fact that the numbers are there at all means *something* is happening. But I want more to happen: I want proof that I'm making the numbers move; they're not just passing over me like clouds.

Being on Weight Watchers is sort of the same way sometimes.

One day at my Weight Watchers check-in, Cindy the weigh-in woman, records my total loss at 24.6 pounds. "Al*most*," she chirps. "Another half pound or so and you'll get your magnet." She means a refrigerator magnet. I have vaguely heard of this: you get a refrigerator magnet after you lose twenty-five pounds. I understand this is not meant to be an incentive so much as it is a little commemoration. That's nice. If I make a derisive snort, it's only in my mind.

For a couple of days I don't think anything of the magnet. Mostly because it's, you know, a *magnet*. And yet as the week goes on I start to keep better track of my food again. I write down everything. When I get hungry between meals I drink V8 juice. All the glasses in my sink become gory with V8 residue. I make it a point not to blow off my workouts all week. I am a good little wretch.

"I get a magnet soon," I tell Leigh when we're out on Saturday night. This is my way of explaining why I don't want to order fries before the kitchen closes at Moody's. We both could use some drunk food but I get a big glass of water instead.

"A *what*?"

"A magnet. From Weight Watchers! For losing twenty-five pounds."

"Good for you," says Leigh. I have been waiting for her to say just that so I can roll my eyes. I am drunker than she is. I roll my eyes and then put my head on the table.

My home scale is plummeting to new lows, I think. Really, the needle seems to be getting nearly sucked backward, as if it's trying to resist the pull of the black hole I am creating with my powerful metabolism. I can feel that underneath all my weight there is an amazing furnace working steadily to consume matter; that deep inside me is a sort of boiler room where gleaming muscle-dappled men in undershirts pull huge levers and crank massive wheels amidst hissing steam, an industrious vision that is glorious and proud without being overtly socialist or homoerotic—no, just an awesome living tableau of efficiency. I stand on the scale and smile enigmatically while the world moves in slow motion all around me.

I am like an energy field, shooting quasars in all directions. And then I'll get a magnet.

When I go to the next meeting I'm a little bit early; there is only one woman ahead of me in line. I can see her membership booklet in her hand and can tell from her chart that she'd joined WW with only about seven pounds to lose. People like her mystify me. I wonder what *she* thinks about getting a magnet.

She gets on the scale and stares down at the digital readout. "Okay," I hear her say to Cindy the weigh-in woman, "I have a question about goal weight? Because I guess I *am* at my goal weight. But actually at my *height* I could have more to go, right? Because, I mean, look at the chart."

More people are getting in line behind me and Our Lady of a Thousand Questions goes on. "So what about Lifetime Membership? That's maintenance, right? And I don't have to pay the weekly fees?" She goes *on and on* as if the loss of seven pounds has created a howling void inside her, a total abyss of sheer inquisitive need. She asks so many questions it gets so I can only *think* in questions. Can Cindy please explain that whole part of the brochure again? And can Cindy please tell her a few anecdotes about other people who have reached their goal weight? And could Cindy congratulate her some more?

All I want to do is experience the mock thrill of Refrigerator Magnet Honor and then go home. I have decided that, yes, it's perfectly okay to want a refrigerator magnet that says I have lost twenty-five pounds. However, I am not going to let this get in the way of my big plans for being very blasé about my magnet. I am so *not* going to chat it up with Cindy when I get it, not like the little hooker in front of me who is being all high maintenance about Maintenance. All I want to do is step on the scale when she's done.

Now Cindy is jotting down my numbers and punching them into her calculator: I've gone down only .2 pounds. I have lost 24.8 pounds.

"Oh!" says Cindy when she sees what has happened. "*Hmm,*" she says.

She writes down the total and hands my booklet back to me but I want to stay right where I am on the scale. I feel like Cindy owes me something somehow. Loudly and very deliberately I say, "Damn!" I want to say something a lot worse: *damn* is nasal, it's Mom Profanity. Even so, I want to say it again, but I know I shouldn't.

I say it again in the car: *Damn!* I probably shouldn't be driving, because I want to hit something. I think I would maybe like to hit a Dumpster. Not hard; just enough to knock it over. That would help, somehow. I want to buy a pack of cigarettes, too, and I want to smoke them until I pass out.

When I was little and had tantrums, part of the rage was always about the fact that the thing denied me was so very *lame*. I have always wanted it known that on the afternoon my screams alarmed the good people of the Benton Harbor KOA campground in 1981, I knew full well that it was *just* an inner tube floating away down the river. Other times, during other rages, it's been *just* a game token or an old T-shirt or a milkshake or a rubber bracelet or a raffle ticket or a Bonne Bell lip gloss. I hate how much they matter. I hate how next I will go to the meeting and Cindy will say something like "Now *there* you go! At *last*."

The next Wednesday I deliberately go to a different Weight Watchers meeting—the 12:30 P.M. one instead of the 5:30. I do this just so Cindy won't have the satisfaction of giving it to me. She would want me to act happy, to babble with gratitude like I'm on a game show. Screw that. Plus I'm going before lunch. Maybe I'm being a little too crafty about it all.

My total loss comes in at 25.2 pounds. They give me

the magnet. It's a blue and yellow star spangled by three little red stars. In the center is a big red 25 and the words *I did it!* floating above. The whole aesthetic is very *Electra Woman and Dyna Girl.* It looks as if I should be able to touch it and have special powers.

Two weeks later I go back to the 5:30 meeting and I watch as the digital scale blinks its way up and back to settle at 202.4. Cindy takes out her calculator again. "Twenty-seven pounds!" she tells me. I nod. "Wait," she says. She opens the cabinet next to the scale and fishes something out of a bag and presents it to me with a big, sweet smile. It's another fucking magnet.

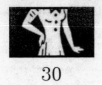

who wears the pants

Nathan says, "If you're going to mention me on your website you're going to have to think up a nickname for me."

"But what about 'The Manatee?' " That's what Sarah calls him on her site.

"No, I hate that. I want something different," he says.

We are waiting for coffee and an order of fried chicken fingers. It seems the Golden Angel Pancake House has become our place. Nathan doesn't like ethnic food. He says he does but I say Italian doesn't count.

"You forgot French," he says. "I like French food."

"I don't think pancakes are French."

"I didn't *order* any pancakes tonight, *okay?*"

"So what do you think of this guy Jared from the Subway commercials?" Nathan asks me. We're on the phone.

"What do you mean? Do I think he lost all that weight

for real?" There are rumors that he didn't really lose two hundred pounds from eating Subway sandwiches, or that he did, but that he gained it all back and that it's his twin brother in the commercials. Or that he had surgery, or a tapeworm. It's all bullshit, I'm sure.

"Like would you date him?"

"What kind of a question is that?"

"Would you?"

"No." There's something about Jared in those commercials, the way he waves at Subway employees from the street, the way they nod back with their yellow visors. I wonder if he's obligated to do that in real life. It makes me glad I'm on the Internet and don't have to go out in public like that to promote *my* amazing weight loss.

"You dig Jared from Subway," Nathan says. "Admit it."

"No way."

"You're *hot* for him. You want to climb into his fat pants with him." Nathan is a little obsessed with Jared's Fat Pants, if you ask me. We've discussed them before, and while he doesn't agree with me, I believe Nathan is actually jealous that he doesn't get to show off Fat Pants as big as Jared's, trousers big enough that a single leg can hold all of the New Jared.

"You could get into the other leg," Nathan says. "And then roll around on the floor with him. You *know* you want to get with Jared."

"You're totally starting to scare me."

I didn't buy grape jelly but I don't get what the problem is.

"First, you never have anything to eat here and then

you don't even get the right stuff to make sandwiches." He is turning the jar of strawberry preserves around and around in his hands as if he could somehow, upon the next rotation, make the label say grape.

"Look, I didn't think about it; I just don't use grape jelly. Sorry."

"Everyone uses grape."

"Dude, I got *bread* for you." He doesn't appreciate what a big deal it is for me to keep bread in my home. *Unfrozen* bread; sliced bread; whole pieces unencumbered from the loaf and ready to throw themselves into the vortex of a 9 P.M. binge.

"Not eating bread is one thing. Not eating *grape jelly* is fucked up."

"No it's not. I can't stand grape-flavored stuff." And now I'm going to have to tell him about how I hate grape flavoring because of a disgusting experience involving a grape Slurpee I consumed when I was six. It came in a big tall cup with a picture of Velma from *Scooby-Doo* on it, and for about a year afterward I regarded Velma from *Scooby-Doo* with great trepidation simply because of what happened later on that night with the grape Slurpee and me. Let's just say that what happened, happened to the bed, too. I tell Nathan the story and he loves it.

"So would the same thing happen if you ate grape jelly now?" he asks. "It would, wouldn't it?"

"Well, no. I just wouldn't like it."

"One of these days I'm going to make you eat grape jelly," he says. "And then tie you to the bed."

"That's mean," I say. After that, whenever he talks

about the Slurpee Incident (which is often), I call him Grape Ape in retaliation.

"Hey, call me that," he says one day. "On your site. My nickname can be Grape Ape."

"What, you like that?"

"Yeah. Call me Grape Ape."

I introduce Grape Ape to my readers, tentatively. First I drop a reference to *this friend of mine*; a week later I mention him by nickname and say, just in passing, that he's my boyfriend. I get a little rush scrolling through the new emails that follow the post. People are writing to say they're happy for me.

"Congratulations!" says Marla, who emails me once a month or so. "He sounds way better than that Little Man guy you wrote about a few months ago."

"I was hoping you'd find someone," says another reader, as if she were my great-aunt or something. Someone else—"Aeon Flux" again—speculates that I might be more open to a relationship now that I've made the decision to "make a change for the better" and "cast off emotional as well as physical weight."

I laugh about it with Sarah that night when I am at their place with Nathan.

"Someone wrote that? Who died and made *her* Dr. Phil?" Sarah asks.

"I know! Apparently only *now* do I have the courage to let a man touch my ass."

"I hate that shit," says Sarah. "Like we're scared because we're fat or something."

Of course, I point out, I reserve the right to be scared for other reasons.

"Of course," says Sarah. "This is *Nathan* we're talking about."

"Hey," Nathan says. "Show me the jeans you wore when you were *really* fat."

He's come over to my place and we're getting ready to go out, but he wants to change first. For a straight guy he's really into clothes; I guess it's because of the weight he's lost.

He is looking through his stash of shirts in my closet. More than once he's gotten himself something new at the Ragstock store across the street from the bookstore and brought it back to my place. He has been working a lot but he takes up space even when he's not here. They're just shirts but each shirt is someplace he's been. So is my apartment; so is my neighborhood, which he hates, because nothing here is ever open late enough for him.

"You need to buy better jeans," he keeps telling me. "The waist is too high on all of them." I tell him I wasn't exactly into wearing that low-rise shit when I was a size 22, which leads to talking about Really Big Fat Pants again, which leads to him wanting to see *my* jeans.

I've already gotten rid of the very biggest stuff, but I have one last pair of jeans that I am hoping I'll never have to wear again. They're from Lane Bryant (their faux-designer "Venezia" store brand), size 20, in a terribly mis-interpreted boot-cut style. They pooch out at the hips; they flare out too much below the knee; the prefaded denim is too stiff. They try hard, so fucking hard, those jeans, but they're stupid and clowny, and all clumsy with wide pylon legs; they're blocky and massive like concrete supports built to hold up your ass like it was the I-94. He holds them up and looks at the pre-frayed cuffs.

"Hmm," he says. "These are almost cool."

"No, they're not," I say.

He is taking off his own jeans and putting on mine. I'm laughing but he goes on buttoning them up. The jeans fit his waist and then hang down everywhere else, just a little, and *just so,* he seems to be thinking. I don't believe it: he is checking himself out in the mirror. He turns from one side to the other.

"Nathan," I say. "You are not going out in my Lane Bryant jeans."

"Why not?" he says. "I like them. Don't they look good?"

"They . . . uh . . ." I look at him. They actually do look sort of okay.

"I don't think I can answer that," I tell him. "Because I know they're my Lane Bryant fat-girl jeans."

"But they look pretty good, right?"

"I guess," I say. Maybe it doesn't matter where they come from. I probably should just accept this: my boyfriend looks good in Lane Bryant jeans.

We go out to Ricochet's, where we meet up with Leigh.

"Know where I got my jeans?" he asks Leigh.

"Um . . . where?"

"Lane Bryant," he says proudly, emphasizing each syllable while I roll my eyes. "Mm-hmm. Lane *Bryant.*"

"I have no response to that," Leigh says.

A few days later I talk to Sarah. "Yeah, so he came home the other night," she says, "and he was all, 'Do you like my jeans? They're *Venezia*.'"

"Oh, Jesus." Now I'll never get them back, though I suppose I *shouldn't* want them back.

"He fucking loves them," says Sarah.

the internet adds 10 pounds

JournalCon Chicago is taking place for an entire weekend at a Days Inn in Lincoln Park. Friday night there's a party at John Barleycorn's, a bar near the hotel, and I meet Sarah at her and Nathan's apartment so we can go together.

Nathan isn't coming along. "You go and meet all your fat fans," he says.

"Shut up," says Sarah. "Wendy and I are fat, too."

"I didn't say you weren't," he says. He gives me a kiss. "Have fun," he says.

Sarah parks her car as close as we can get to the bar, which is in the middle of one of the more relentlessly trendy north side neighborhoods. Packs of girls in their twenties pass us on the street hugging their own arms for warmth;

it's fifty degrees out but they're wearing tube tops and halters and tiny cap sleeves.

"They're going to die," I say, after a group of them pass us.

"Just a few. Thinning the herd," says Sarah.

I worry a little about where we are. "We're geeks here," I tell Sarah, though I mean that in a good way. Across the street is a beer garden seething with frat guys.

Sarah nods. "You've met people from the Internet before, right?" she asks. "I mean, besides me and Lexy."

I think about the trip to Las Vegas. "Yeah. That was all right. Except for the part when I got back and found out how fat I was."

"That won't be a problem this time," Sarah says.

"I guess not," I say. I know she means that it'll be different because I've lost thirty pounds. But there are other reasons, too.

We edge past the crowds waiting outside the bars on Lincoln Avenue. This isn't really my world at all; we're going to an outpost of another world, one I've worked hard on being a part of, where my weight is the first thing anyone knows about me. I guess my fat is there whether I show up or not.

The JournalCon group is in a private party room at the bar. Sarah and I stand at the door and look in.

"They look okay to you?" Sarah asks.

There are about twenty people milling around. The only thing that immediately strikes me as odd about the group is that two people have colored hair. I mean there's one woman with pink hair and another with bright red. Otherwise, though, everyone looks pretty normal. To be honest, it's only the two dye jobs that convince me we're in the right room, since nobody with hair like that would be caught in John Barleycorn's under normal circumstances.

"They look fine," I say, and it's true. We walk in.

Someone waves at us from across the room. I'm pretty sure it's one of the JournalCon organizers. Her name is Jessamyn and her picture is on the front page of her site. Sarah and I wonder how people are going to know who we are, since Sarah doesn't have photos of herself on her site and I only have weird, anonymous karaoke shots. But then I see two girls who are pointing in my direction. They're looking at my Television Without Pity shirt.

"I think they've just figured out who you are," Sarah says. The girls are coming up to me; one of them actually sort of *hustles* over with her arm reaching out as if to pet me. "Oh, my God, *Poundy!*" she's saying.

"I'm Wendy," I tell her, nodding.

"I know," she says. "Poundy!"

I want to correct her but I'd hate how I'd sound if I did that. The girl has a convention badge that indicates her name is Rachel and her online journal is called Mischief. The other girl is named Caitlyn, whose site is called Clever Clever.

"You look *great!*" Caitlyn says, as if to congratulate me for something.

"You really do," Rachel agrees. And here all I did was show up.

*   *   *

Once Sarah and I are given badges with our names and websites on them we start moving slowly through the room to see who's here. I see badges for weblogs and journals I've heard of—Darn Tootin', terriblyhappy.com, Glitter—as well as for sites I don't know at all. I'm not sure whether it's better to make eye contact with a person and *then* look at their badge, or if it's acceptable to do it the other way.

A guy in a gray hooded sweatshirt keeps hanging out near us. He has long black hair and a goatee. His badge says his name is "Kristofer" and he has four sites listed: one with a Diaryland.com address; two at Livejournal.com; and another at Diary-X.com. He never introduces himself but when I find myself floating on the periphery of all the conversations in the room I try small talk with him.

"Wow, four sites," I say. "Are they all your journals?"

"They are all my writings," he says.

"Okay. And they're all different?"

He points to one. "This one is for my fictional works," he explains. "Originally it was for my novella but I had to take that down."

"Why?"

"It was very dark. Very much about the darker side of reality."

"And people couldn't handle that?" I'm trying to guess here.

"I created another journal for all my works of darkness. Because I write so much about that." He goes on to tell me about the journal he has just for his dreams as well as the

one he has for his poetry, which is often "about madness."
"Mental illness is very dark, too," he says.

"I'm sure it is," I tell him.

"I have it, you know."

"Wow. What kind?"

"Because this guy stabbed me last year! He, like, stabbed me right here!" He clutches his upper arm.

"*Wow*. I'm sorry. Why'd he do that?"

"He was against me. He still is. I have to be careful."

"Wow."

"I'm on disability now."

"Because of the stabbing?"

"No. The mental illness. You know?"

Nobody seems to be coming up and joining our conversation for some reason.

I can tell that a lot of people here met at last year's Journal-Con; they race across the room to hug each other.

The most popular person here seems to be a guy named Rob, who, according to Jessamyn, has had an online journal since 1997. Since he started writing he'd moved from the Midwest to the East Coast, changed jobs at least four times, got engaged, married, and had a daughter. "Yeah," Jesssamyn says. "He had this Rob for President campaign a couple years ago, and all these people were putting up buttons on their own sites."

"He was kidding, right?" I ask.

"Oh, yeah. But still." Rob seems to have three or four people hovering around him all the time. I might as well hover, too.

"So I'm totally standing here being this Rob fan," says an older woman near me. "I'm not even being ironic about it."

"I just want to say hi to him," I say. "I just started reading his journal." Or I plan to. In fact I want to run home and look up all the websites of everyone here, all the blogs and online journals. Before I came here I visited only a few of them; now I feel a little like I haven't studied for a test.

The woman looks at my badge: "Oh, you're the girl who does Poundy."

"That's me, all right." My badge says *Pound,* but, well, okay.

"Wow. You know, I guess I expected you to be much heavier," she says.

I nod. I guess that's a compliment.

I wish I'd brought a camera. People are bringing out their digital cameras and asking each other to take their pictures; they pose together and wave other people over to join the shot. Mischief Rachel offers to email me a photo she took of me and Sarah.

"I might put it up on my weblog, too, if that's okay," she says. "I bet people are going to want to know what you really look like."

"Well, I do have those progress pictures on my site," I point out.

"Yeah, that's true," says Rachel. "But I mean pictures of you in person. That's different, you know?"

*   *   *

I'm talking with a woman named Amy who says, "By the way? My good friend Ericka is *obsessed* with your site. She loves it. She actually told me to stalk you tonight."

"Thank you," I say, "I think."

I look at Amy hard, and she looks like she would tell me if her friend was planning on showing up at my workplace with a giant doll she'd made to resemble me.

"I think she follows your site more closely than mine," she says. "Anyway, she wants proof that I'd talked to you."

"Really? Like an autograph?" I say. Oh God, an *autograph*? I sound like an asshole.

But Amy has a better idea, which is for us to pose for a picture with a little sign that reads HI ERICKA! written in Sharpie marker on one of the paper plates from the snack table. I hold up the plate and wave at whoever the moment's for.

I find Sarah by herself at the bar. "It's too bad neither of us are looking to hook up," she says. "There are actually some decent-looking guys at this thing."

"Are you having a good time?"

She nods. "I'm not all that into it." She doesn't seem to like big groups all that much. "But don't worry about me. I know it's different for you."

"It's weird," I tell her. In the past hour I have spoken with people I know only as: Lady Grey, Scruple.net, Melinda P., WeetzieBat, and Bugger. More than once someone saw my name on my badge and then looked me up and down to see how fat I was.

*   *   *

The girl with dyed bright-red hair seems clever and a little mean. Usually she has a small crowd around her, too, but at the moment she's just standing by one of the tables near the wall.

I look down at her badge: *Dana*, it says. Her site is Bobofett.com and she's come all the way from Connecticut.

"My site has nothing to do with *Star Wars*," she says.

I nod. "I don't think that's how you spell Boba Fett anyway."

"How would you know? Are you one of those *Star Wars* fans?" she asks.

"Um, no," I say.

"Good. Hey, I saw you talking to Count Kookula," she says.

"Oh, that Kristofer guy?"

"He's my *favorite person here*." She grins.

Day Two of JournalCon convenes in the lobby of the Days Inn. Everyone appears to be at least a little hungover.

"Where'd you go off to last night?" Rachel asks. I'd left with Sarah to be with Nathan, though since he's been working the closing shift at the bookstore, most of our time together is spent asleep.

"Oh, we thought maybe you guys had gone off with Count Kookula," says Dana. Nobody knows where Kristofer went. He'd never booked a room.

I hear snippets about late-night parties in some of the rooms. Lauren of pinkcadillac.net held back Rachel's hair while she threw up. The guy with the site called Squeeze-box was supposedly caught in the bathroom with Jessica G., but it remains to be seen whether it's an actual scandal or just a joke.

Kristofer is found asleep on a couch at the far end of the meeting room where we'll have our panel discussions. Sarah and I walk in there first with Jessamyn, but when we see him we all hang back near the door.

He has left a note on the table: "I am resting. If some-one would like to take a picture of me in my shroud and send it to me later, I would appreciate it."

"His *shroud?*" Sarah whispers. We can see he is lying on his back in solemn repose with his sweatshirt hood up.

"He can't stay here," Jessamyn hisses. "If he's spent the night here we could get in trouble with the hotel."

We look across the room again and see him sit bolt up-right like a rigor mortis corpse.

"Let's go. Now," Sarah says. "Oh, shit, hurry."

My cell phone rings when we've just broken for lunch. "So how's the Fat Chicks Convention?" Nathan wants to know.

"Stop calling it that," I say.

"Have you given your big motivational speech yet? With all the fabulous diet tips?"

I hand the phone to Sarah. "Your roommate's being to-tally obnoxious," I tell her.

We're at a Chinese restaurant. "We're going to order some dim sum to share," says a girl at my table whose name I don't even know. "Can you eat that?" she asks, looking at me. "Like are you in a mood to cheat this weekend? I bet you are, huh?"

A group of us are back in the Days Inn lobby when we notice a notebook on a table right near the meeting room door. It's Kristofer's.

"Oh my God," Caitlyn whispers. She goes over and picks it up. She opens it up and starts flipping through the pages.

"HE'S RIGHT BEHIND YOU!" Rachel yells, just for fun.

For dinner the whole group goes to a tapas restaurant where we take up four big tables. Sarah wants to sit at the same table as one of the guys she'd noticed the other night. "Oh my God, I've been staring at him all day. You know how I told you I have this thing for guys with shaved heads? He's the kind of guy I'm talking about."

The guy with the shaved head is from New York State, Sarah finds out, and his name is Dan. Everyone else at the table is sort of quiet and shy, myself included.

There is sangria; there are marinated mushrooms and crab cakes and dates wrapped in bacon, and it all tastes wonderful but I don't want to take a lot; I don't feel quite right here. It would have helped if I'd spent the night before in the hotel with everyone else. I am looking around at the other tables. That girl Rachel is kneeling on her chair and laughing hard. Somebody made stickers for their website and Caitlyn is sticking one on her sweater. Three girls who met at the first JournalCon are just coming in from getting tattoos together; a couple of them are pulling back their gauze bandages and letting others take a peek.

All these people are real; somehow I hadn't expected that. They require conversation, and attention, and real food that at another time I might have kept eating until I was able to feel happy. Now I think I should leave it for the people who are really *here*.

After a while the waiters stop bringing new dishes and start taking away old ones, and people begin getting up to visit the bar and the other tables. Dana, the girl with the bright-red hair and the non–*Star Wars* site, is ahead of me waiting for the bathroom.

"He's gone," she says.

"Who?"

"The Kook. Kristofer," she says. "He left before dinner. He said he was going to the bus station."

"Aww," I say. I feel a little bad. I heard he'd wanted to perform a special reading of one of his journal entries, complete with dimmed lights, but the JournalCon organizers had claimed there wasn't enough time.

"Yeah, poor Kook," Dana says. She looks around. "Okay. So before I came here I said something on my site about how I was going to be fatter in person—like, a joke, you know? Or, really, not a joke because, hey . . ." She motions toward herself. "I guess I just didn't want people to expect someone thinner than I am."

I nod. She's about my size.

"So then," she says, "see that chick over there?" She points over at a woman named Kate. "She came up to me

and she said, 'You know, I read your site, and you're right—
you *are* fatter in person.' I mean, *what the hell?*"

"Come sing karaoke with us," Sarah says. By *us* she means
the whole group, but I can't help but notice that she and
this guy Dan are sticking together.

"I don't know. I might go back to your place," I tell her.
Nathan gets off work soon.

"Nathan won't be home until after eleven-thirty," she
says. "Come on."

I'm not staying long. The Hidden Cove Lounge is
packed, and I can tell it'll take forever for the people in our
group to sing. I stand near the bar and watch. Rachel
comes over and joins me while we watch a burly guy—not
from our group—sing "Night and Day."

"So you're singing, right? If you want I can take some
pictures," she says.

"Thanks, but I'm actually a pretty crappy singer," I tell
her.

"Yeah, but, you know, you have those pictures from
Vegas," she says. "It would be really cool if there were pictures of you singing karaoke and this time you were thinner . . ." Her voice trails off. "Don't you think?"

"Yeah, that would be great," I say. "I'm just not up to it
tonight." I feel guilty for not feeling the difference every
moment.

"Are you leaving?" Sarah asks. "You're going to miss me
sing 'Like A Virgin.' "

"Sorry," I say, though I'm pretty sure this guy Dan is not

going to miss her performance. The night is getting weirder.

"Oh, don't go," says Kate, the girl who told Dana she was fatter in person.

"I have to," I tell her. "I'm meeting up with my boyfriend."

"Well, tell *Grape Ape* I said hello," she says. She says it bemusedly, the way you might ask about Mrs. Claus when you visit Santa at the mall.

"I thought you'd be out later," Nathan says.

"I missed you," I tell him.

His bed is pushed up against the wall and I have to climb over him to get to the side I usually sleep on.

"Watch out for the ashtray," he says. His bed is a futon on a metal frame near the floor and his room isn't much bigger than the bed. I manage to make it over without stepping on him or anything important and lie down.

"You came back to be with me?" he says.

"Well, yeah," I tell him.

He's hogging the one good quilt so I rummage around for something to sleep under. He has mismatched flannel sheets, two grayish, pilling blankets, a small afghan, and a kid's sleeping bag that he uses as a comforter sometimes. To be honest, I don't think I'd want to go near his bed if he wasn't in it.

I pull the sleeping bag up to my chin and find the edge that doesn't have a zipper, and I curl up against him spoon-style.

"So were you a total celebrity there?" he asks.

"I don't know," I say. "Sort of. Not really." I think for a moment. "They're nice people and it was okay. But I didn't feel like myself there."

I press against his back and try to match my breathing to his. This might help.

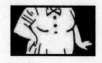

chickenfinger

At the Lincoln Restaurant Nathan orders some pancakes and a big chef salad.

"I didn't eat all day," he says.

"Wow. What happened?" I ask.

"Nothing. I just decided not to eat today," he says. "I'm trying to lose these ten pounds."

Apparently, there have been ten pounds. I didn't know there were ten, but then, for that matter I didn't know they were his, either. I thought it was just the feeling I was getting from all this diner food.

"So you're having this one meal? At the *Lincoln?*" Behind us is a glass case full of pies, the kind trimmed with whipped cream gone gummy from being chilled for two days.

"Yep," he says.

We keep doing this: going to the Lincoln or the Golden

Angel or even the Le Sabre, where Nathan either has chicken fingers for breakfast at 2 P.M. when he wakes up after a closing shift at the bookstore, or else he has breakfast at 8 P.M. after a day shift. I'm on his schedule on weekends, staying up until 3 A.M. in order to spend time with him after work and then sleeping in until the afternoon. I feel like I live underwater.

"That's not the best way to do it, I don't think," I tell him when our food comes and he reaches for the syrup.

"It's how I did it before," he says.

"Well, you think maybe I know a little something about how to do all this, too?"

"Actually, no," he says. "No, you don't." There's a snort in his voice; he's *kidding*. In the first few weeks my impulse was to laugh back at it. Then I laughed so much I thought I sounded nervous and suddenly developed an opposite response. Now I don't know what my reflexes are. At any time I could kick or I could stay still.

"What do you mean I don't?"

"I mean, look at your site," he says. "When's the last time you mentioned losing any weight?"

"At least I *do* the right things," I say. I can't believe how I sound.

"Yeah, but where does it get you? You can be all 'you go, girl' if it makes you feel better, but I'm going to do it my way," he says. He is trying very concertedly not to finish his pancakes; playing with the top one and folding it back until it falls apart in wet pieces. "I'm going to try and ride my bike this weekend. There's this trail that goes almost to

Northbrook. Twenty miles I think. I did it a couple times last year."

"You know, you look fine to me," I tell him.

"Yeah, thanks," he says. His voice is flat.

"What?"

"I mean, maybe it's fine for *you*."

Sarah broke up with Josh. "It's not because of that guy Dan," she says, but then she admits that, well, in a way it was, because if things had been going okay she wouldn't have let that night with Dan happen.

We're sitting in her and Nathan's living room and smoking and waiting for Nathan to come home so we can watch a movie.

"What was going on with you and Josh?" I ask.

"Nothing all that wrong," she says. "He just wasn't right. It was like the more he *tried* to be right, the more stunted he got." She grabs the ashtray and brings it over. "The weird thing is that I got an email from Dan the other day."

"Are you going to write him back?"

"Yeah. I mean, I did," she says. She has this strange look. "I don't know. I don't know what I think. It's not because of Dan. Dan's in New York."

"Sarah was looking up airfares," Nathan says later. "I saw that she was visiting travel websites."

"You think she's going to visit that guy?"

"Whatever," he says. "She's nuts. Every day I'm glad I'm not still dating her."

Sometimes it feels like that first night at the Yankee Clipper, where he's teasing me and I'm taking it and I'm laughing along because I feel like this is all a prelude to something. I worry that this is all there is. And then I seem to have forgotten how to do everything else in my life. When I read over my Weight Watchers brochures they say I have to "keep track of how many points are in the things I eat" and then sometimes "not eat" too much of some things and also "work out" on "a regular basis."

No, really, I think; what do I have to *do*?

"You haven't updated your site this week," says Krista, one of my regular readers. "But I bet that's because you're all happy with The Guy."

That's the story, I suppose.

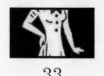

you take the good, you take the bad

Am I freaking you out? Ericka writes. She keeps typing line after line:

Seriously.

Let me know if I flip you out.

Or get too intense or something.

I really am that big of a fan.

It's one thing to get an email from someone like Ericka. It's another to experience her in instant message chat, to see the enthusiasm ticking out in real time.

I feel like I'm burning WW Points just TALKING to you!

This is so cool! HI!

Am I typing too much?

Are we best friends yet?

I hope it's okay that I gave her my screen name.

*   *   *

Ericka has been writing me on and off for over a year. After her friend Amy had her picture taken with me at Journal-Con this past fall I searched through my inbox for emails from her. Reading them all at once was a little unnerving.

"It's Ericka AGAIN," she'd written last February. "Because I can't leave you alone."

In April she wrote, "This has to be the fourth or fifth time I've written you. I'M NOT EVEN KIDDING."

After JournalCon: "Oh, oh, oh, my God. Amy sent me the picture. Thank you!!!"

Last week she wrote: "My screen name is 'Crikes6' on AOL. I know you probably can't give out yours because you are ALL HOT. HOTT, even, with the extra Heavy Metal T. But feel free to say hi if you're ever on."

Yesterday she wrote, "I know you write back because you're nice, but really, don't worry about me. I just write you a lot because that's how I am. Really, just ignore me."

Ericka is about my age—early thirties—and she lives in Crystal Lake, Illinois. I find it on the back of my Chicago map, on the side that shows the far, far suburbs. She says it takes about two hours to drive to the city from where she is.

"So I'm not going to just turn up on your front steps, if you were wondering," she says.

She has a husband and a daughter, Keegan, aged two. She talks about someplace called Gymboree and I think once she may have used the word *scrapbook* as a verb. I can't say I know her world very well.

"You do NOT sell Mary Kay," I say, when she tells me what she does.

"No shit, I do," she types back. "I just started."

"Wow. Well, I guess you can make good money. I've heard. I mean, I've read," I say. I imagine her in a pink power suit lugging a cosmetics case the size of an ottoman. I can't believe she reads my site.

She says, "I can tell you don't appreciate Mary Kay for the completely demented makeup sorority that it is. So I will not even tell you about the crazy CANDLELIGHT CEREMONY that I had to go through. And the GIANT TACKYASS RHINESTONE COCKTAIL RING that I'll get once I sell to 30 people."

"No way. Tell me!" I type, because if Ericka's not nuts, she's my spiritual twin. I suppose she could be both.

The next night we spend two hours talking—or typing, or whatever—about the TV show *The Facts of Life*. Ericka has many pop culture obsessions, especially about that show.

We discuss how Natalie got a bad rep as the "fat chick" on the show when really, the rest of the cast (except Jo) caught up with her in a few seasons, puffing up stealthily, almost imperceptibly, until sometime in 1987 when suddenly they were lurching around in gigantic, boxy blazers. It stands to reason that a show that would put a girl on roller skates for a whole season to make her taller would drown three young women in shoulder pads to make them seem smaller.

"They looked good though," says Ericka. "In their own way."

We find out we both had the same shameful thought whenever Natalie had a love interest on the show, which was to suspect that the guy who got cast to play her boyfriend probably got flak from his buddies at Performing Arts High School.

"It was these sidelong glances she'd give him," says Ericka. "You could tell she didn't like him, either."

We decide that our fascination with Natalie has to do with her bizarre predicament: she was dumpy and awkward enough to sit at our lunch tables with us and yet she was trapped on a famous TV show for years and years and years. We were glad she was there on screen but we didn't want to *be* her.

"She runs just like me," says Ericka. "I saw it on the episode where they all go to Australia. She runs to pick up a boomerang and she sort of lumbers along with her arms hanging at her sides. It's just so sad."

We consider how you could never say the title of the show without the sense you were saying the *Fats of Life*.

"They really were the Fats of Life," says Ericka. "They never had Very Special Episodes about being fat."

"It's true, they didn't."

"They just were, and that was life," says Ericka.

"So are you okay with my crazy slobbering fan shit?" she asks.

I tell her I'm used to it now but that I don't understand it.

"I really am exaggerating a little bit. This is just how I am," she says.

She hits RETURN and then takes a long time to type the next part.

> *It's just that last year I was ready EVERY SINGLE DAY to step in front of a bus. Because I felt horrible about myself and the way that I looked. I had NO CONTROL and it scared me. I saw a picture of me after I had Keegan where I was 270 pounds and it was like getting slapped in the face. I found your site and it helped so so much to read you because you seemed like someone just like me. And you were doing all this stuff so I did it, too.*

I take in everything she's said. "So you've been losing some weight, then?"

"I've lost 125 pounds," she writes. "Since I started reading your site, like a year ago or so."

First I type, WHAT? and then I delete it. I write, "Oh my God." I had no idea.

She says she did Weight Watchers and she walked a lot. I pull up a couple of her old emails. "I just got the special keychain for 50 pounds," she says in one of them. I can't believe I missed this.

"I get kind of obsessed with stuff though," she says. "I bet you can tell. I really got into it."

I want her to tell me how that happened. I want to catch whatever she has.

"But I wouldn't have in the first place if I didn't see that you were doing it. And that you weren't trying to be all perfect about it. And that you didn't care too much about it sometimes, even though I know that probably you really do."

*   *   *

"I need to tell you that I'm jealous," I write her. "You did way more than I think I'll ever do. My God."

"You would have done it if you needed to," she writes.

"Yeah, well, I'm still over 200 pounds," I remind her.

"That's not really what I mean," she says.

#

and

Once, a couple of years ago, I was walking down the street and some guy in a passing car yelled out that I was fat. Really, though, he just shouted "FAT!" out the window.

There wasn't a lot of traffic. I was the only person on the sidewalk on this block. It was a sunny afternoon and a station wagon went by and this shitty little transaction took place. There was no "you," and no verb; there are parts of a sentence that have to do with the state of being, but I didn't hear them as the car passed.

I didn't know what I was supposed to do next. I tried to think of something to yell back. I could only come up with "And . . .?"

And then I kept walking, because it seemed the thing to do. I wasn't sure, but it seemed that it was what anyone would do.

The truth about me used to be out loud like that; it

used to have a name and sometimes when it was called out I'd be walking along, wondering if anyone else heard it and thought it meant me.

Now it seems like I can never get outside the truth, and I can't hear it, at least not between each breath.

34

your stuff

It needs to be said that we're not breaking up.

"I think I'm going to be bringing some of your stuff back tonight," I tell Nathan. "Is there anything you need right now?"

"Need what?" he says. He's finally called me back from work. I can hear Bookstore Jazz tootling in the background.

"Your stuff. You've got a lot of stuff at my place right now, and when I come over I thought I'd bring some of it. We're still on for tonight, right?" These days I have to ask. He's working a lot and I never seem to know when his nights off are.

"Yeah, sure," he says.

"So if there's anything in particular you need, just let me know and I'll bring it."

"Like what?" he says.

"I don't know. Anything. Like something you might

have left among all your stuff and that you might want, since you haven't been here in a while." Two and a half weeks. We've been dating three months, which means that more than 16 percent of our relationship has been this weird interval of Non-Stuff-Visitation on his part and curatorial duties on mine.

"*Something?*" he says, sort of suspiciously. "Can you give me a hint?"

"Wait, no. I'm not trying to hint. Just that . . . I don't know. Your *tapes?* Do you want your Andy Kaufman tapes? Because we watched them all and they're still here."

"Okay. Yeah. And there are a couple shirts, I guess. Thanks."

"No problem."

"So what's all this supposed to mean anyway?" he says. I didn't think he'd ask.

"*Nothing.*" We're not breaking up. "Nothing, okay? Really. Sorry, it's just that my place is a mess and I haven't seen you and—"

"I know," he says. "God, I didn't really think that."

"Good." I hate him for kidding about that.

"Though it's weird that you'd think I *would,*" he says.

It's Saturday and Sarah's gone for the weekend. She's flown to New York to visit Dan. "It's crazy," she'd told me. I couldn't believe it either.

"It's something she's got to do, I guess," Nathan had said.

"You think?" Nathan usually wouldn't miss a chance to call Sarah a flake.

"Absolutely," he'd said.

Anyway, Sarah's away, which is why nobody is there to tell me where Nathan is an hour after he said he'd be home, after he said he'd call and I'd come over.

Nathan doesn't have a cell phone. "Hey," I tell his voice-mail at work, "you're probably not there, since it's midnight and the store's been closed for an hour, and it's Saturday night, which I mention only because I'm sure you'll be—I mean, I *hope* you'll be—hearing this message long after the fact," I say. I wonder how my voice is going to come across when he hears this. "The fact being that, well, I don't know where you are." I was supposed to hear from him two hours ago now. I don't like how I sound.

I have a bag full of his things so I have a purpose here. It's really just an errand I'm running here, at 12:30 A.M., driving down to Bucktown to drop off some stuff for my boyfriend, who has probably just fallen asleep after a long day; who is not answering the phone but will hear the doorbell; whose movements all night have unwittingly fallen into some off-rhythm, some pattern synchronized to just miss hearing the phones ring at work and at home; I imagine a sort of map, a floor plan, a clever cross-section diagram like in those fucking *Family Circus* cartoons with a meandering dotted line showing Nathan's path and all the little accidents of timing and that he encounters at work and home and the space in between, and if I could only see it would make sense and it would be funny even.

I know things just didn't work out tonight but why not drop this stuff off, I mean, as long as I am awake and fully dressed and have a car and know the way to his house, since I completely understand that events simply conspired against Nathan and me spending time together, and instead of trying to fight these forces I'm in my car heading down Western, in the general direction of his neighborhood. I might happen to encounter him on his bike, coming back from Flash Taco, maybe, where it was crowded and took forever to grab a late dinner, or the gas station where he had to fix his tire, returning from some province of reasonable explanation, and it'll be okay, because I'm not fighting this. I won't fight and I'll just relax (he always tells me I need to relax) and I'll manage to crack the code of this whole night. I'll sit on the front steps for an hour until the universe understands I'm here under the most casual circumstances and that we're not breaking up.

I wish Sarah was home. I wish their downstairs neighbors were awake so that I could leave this bag of stuff with them to give to Nathan. I check my voicemail at home again. I just need to give him this stuff, these tapes and shirts and CDs and a bike lock and three books that I'm not going to read after all because I just don't go for the French surrealist shit, sorry, though I am still reading the totally depressing Nathanael West novel he lent me. But the other things aren't me; they shouldn't be lying around in little stacks in my apartment, reminding me that he hasn't been there in forever and that we're out of sync. I just need to get this stuff back to him so that we'll be normal again.

I can't bring myself to just leave the bag by the door. I brought cigarettes. It's cold enough for gloves but I'm smoking with bare hands that I want badly to wash.

Whenever I finish a cigarette I walk to the curb to drop the butt in the gutter and watch for Nathan's bike down the street. I think we're trying to be ourselves again, and I want to give him these things that are his, and then I haven't really thought about what's going to happen next. For now I leave a note telling him I'm glad he hasn't been killed. I ought to start with him being alive and then go from there, I think.

I take the bag with me and get in my car and drive home. It's 1:45 in the morning. I take Milwaukee over to Western. I'm just to Fullerton when my cell phone rings and lights up with his home number.

"Yeah, I'm home now," he says.

"Where the hell were you?!" I yell.

"At *work*."

"I tried calling you there."

"I know," he says. "I was in the back."

"But you knew I called?"

"I don't know. Did you?"

"I . . . *yes*." I guess it's all a mistake.

"Sorry. I didn't mean to be this late," he says. "I didn't think you'd still want to come over."

"Well, I tried to drop off some stuff. But you weren't there and I'm really fucking pissed you didn't call before. I'm on my way home now and I'm going to bed." He worked late, and I tried to stop by, and it's just that the whole night curdled and the hours careened off in different directions, and there's nothing we have to talk about. "Just call me tomorrow, okay?" I wait for him to say something. "*Okay?*"

"I think you need to come back over now," he says. "If you're not too far."

"You want me to come back to your place?"

I'm about a mile away. I'm still on the stretch of Western Avenue south of the expressway. There are all the Mexican restaurants and little bars that I've noticed every time I drive down here; places I don't know a thing about but thought maybe he'd show me. Lots of pink and orange neon signs, plenty of night cheer.

"I think you probably should come back over," he repeats. "It won't take long."

"What won't?"

"I'll meet you downstairs," he says, and hangs up.

back to ourselves

"Tell me what happened," says Michael. It's 6 A.M.; I got home from Nathan's at around 4 A.M. I'd smoked too many cigarettes to sleep easily and I'd laid in bed watching the clock and waiting for it to be a reasonable hour on the East Coast. "I mean, you broke up, but what did he say?"

"Just that he didn't think we meshed that well together."

"Weren't you telling me the same thing about him a couple weeks ago?" Michael asks.

"Yes," I say, but I still want to cry. "He also said . . ." I have to stop and take a breath so I won't lose my shit. "Yeah, he said that he didn't think he should be dating someone else with, um, a . . ."

"Website?"

"No, a 'weight problem.' " I say it that way because I

can't stand that term. Dogs can be said to have weight problems; dogs, and maybe child actors. Not *people*.

"And he said that when he's unhappy he gets fat, and he didn't want to get fat again, and he thought he would if he stayed with me." A hundred or so women seem to think I have something to do with their weight loss; apparently, now I am also responsible for how much a retail manager in Wicker Park weighs. When in the hell did I get more power over other people's fat than my own?

"What a dick," Michael says.

I'm still trying to take it all in. Nathan told me a lot of things and I'm making myself recall everything now so that it doesn't just hit me when I go to bed and wake up again.

"Oh, and he also might have sort of left me for someone else."

It was a girl he works with at the store. Or it wasn't really the girl, Nathan had said, because she was about to go abroad for a semester, but it was the principle of the thing, which he'd started thinking about when Sarah dumped Josh and decided to fly across the country to visit this guy Dan. Nathan listened to Sarah say that no matter what happened in New York she'd be glad she pursued this feeling she'd had; this sense that she was about to find something much better. Nathan had decided to do the same thing. So really, he dumped me for just the *idea* of someone else. That's the part I have to get used to the most.

"Really, ultimately, this is the best thing," says Michael.

"I know."

"And I think maybe you really wanted a boyfriend right now," he says. "As much as you don't like to admit that kind of thing."

"I don't want people to think I'm insecure."

"I know," Michael says.

"Because I hate people assuming that I am."

I've always felt one of the worst things a person could think about me was that I couldn't prevail over my own body, that in addition to my fat I had some poverty of self-worth; I hate the thought that I'm just some kind of Russian nesting doll with the big outside and inevitably, rattling around under all the layers, a crude little peg with a face is the truth of me.

Also the truth is that at this moment I'm crying about being alone on New Year's. It's a week before Thanksgiving right now. "This is the worst time to break up with someone," I say. "Worst fucking time ever."

"Go to sleep," Michael says, "and when you wake up, get online and look up airfares to Raleigh-Durham."

On Thanksgiving Day I decide to put my web journal on hiatus. I don't feel like posting the same stuff I did last year about the holidays, about counting points and bravely resisting sugar cookies.

"A year ago, the only obligation I felt was to write journal entries where I figured out something new," I write. "There are still new things, but I think I need time right now to experience them."

I wonder if anyone can tell that it means I've broken up with Nathan and I'm not quite ready to discuss it.

I read in Sarah's journal that the trip to see Dan went well. Likewise Dan has written on his website about Sarah. Everything went so well that they're spending Christmas together; he's flying out to Chicago to visit her and then they're driving back to upstate New York. She writes that she doesn't think she can be without him now. At least twice a week now she posts long, almost breathless journal entries about taking chances and following convictions and being in love. They are exuberant and real and I can't bring myself to read them.

I email her to say I'm happy for her and I don't ask about Nathan.

Christmas night I'm getting ready to go home, collecting my presents in a shopping bag, and my mother is sitting in the dining room with our cousins, and when I pass by she waves me over. I go to kiss her, because I'm leaving, but instead of saying good-bye she says I look wonderful.

I hug her. "Thank you."

"I can really tell," she says. I know she can tell. I don't know what to do except thank her—thank my mom, though that seems wrong somehow.

She says, "No really, I am telling you," and her eyes are happy. Her left eye never quite aligns with the right; it's a little more pronounced when she's tired. To me, it's always looked like she uses her left eye for thinking; now, she's smiling even with that eye.

I hug her again and then I hang in there a moment and it's hard to step away and it's hard that I have to go. So I tell her it hasn't been easy and she says, "*I know.*"

I can feel my face starting to draw up tight and I don't want to cry. I don't want to cry until I figure out what it's for.

"Merry Christmas," my mom says, and I go.

There's a magazine called *Self*. I've bought the January issue to read on the flight to North Carolina. It's the *Special New Year Body* issue, where there are three full pages devoted to the results of a survey conducted in order to determine American women's feelings about their bodies.

I have the window seat on the plane, which is mostly a good thing. I edge into the short row and buckle myself in long before I have to. The seats to the left of me fill in, though I never really look at the people next to me. I never feel like I'm supposed to, though I notice, in the tight rows, all the different things people do to fold themselves in, so many configurations of bent legs and arms held close. I always feel better when the plane takes off and the noise fills in and dulls the awkwardness.

According to *Self*, forty-two percent of women are satisfied with their body right now. And sixty percent of women say they're happier in their relationships when they're happier with their body. All this concern about "happiness" used to seem kind of stupid to me. I think I used to feel exempt from the question.

Sixty-eight percent of women who *don't* exercise say they are unhappy with their body, but then the nine percent of the women who *are* happy with their body and who do exercise do so only because the media influences them, which means they may not be really happy, or else happy for the wrong reasons.

Eventually, I can see the lights on the ground. It's almost night and everything has given way to rows and patterns and clusters of lights, thousands of them, for buildings and cars and all the places in between lit at intervals. When we land I'll get out and be back in it; I'll join the one hundred percent of whatever.

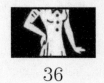

do right

Caitlyn says I'll love her gym, which is a very nice gym, which is in a neighborhood I can't quite afford: a-walk-down-the-street-in-your-cute-clothes-and-run-into-your-cool-friends-at-the-outdoor-café-saying-*Oh, hello!* kind of neighborhood. I get to Women's Workout World by walking through a parking lot; here I feel like I walk through a movie that everyone else but me is in, a movie called *Isn't Life Fabulous*.

When I get there I see the gym is most definitely part of that movie. It's called Cheetah, just the one word in the singular form. More than once I've heard people say, "Oh, I'm meeting so-and-so at *Cheetah*," and I thought they were talking about a restaurant or the kind of bar where there is lots of stainless steel and giant sculpted silver lips as wall sconces.

I suppose I'm part of the movie, too: I'm meeting a

friend here. I hadn't talked to Caitlyn much at JournalCon but we'd met up for drinks a few weeks ago. We'd talked about web journal gossip (word had gotten out about Sarah and Dan, and Caitlyn wanted to hear the details) and weight stuff.

I don't know exactly when I required a slight beer buzz to really talk seriously about Weight Watchers, but I find that it helps.

"I feel *so* good when I do it consistently," I was telling Caitlyn. "Like my body is so in tune with . . . stuff." I lit a cigarette. "And it's weird, but I enjoy cigarettes a lot more," I told her.

"Definitely," Caitlyn said. She lit one, too.

"And I went to weigh in last week and lost, like, a pound and a half." I took a long drag that made my shoulders settle. I liked how right I felt like this. I have been doing well lately.

At Cheetah there's a juice bar café on the ground floor where you can get smoothies and salads; there's three computers where you can get on the Internet, there's exposed brick and polished hardwood and track lighting; the whole place looks designed to make working out seem like a pleasant afterthought, like maybe you were sipping your tea and checking your email when all of a sudden you decided to wander over and, oh, hey, do the StairMaster for forty-five minutes.

They have towel service here. They have dry towels that you get at the door and then neatly rolled damp towels stacked up in a small refrigerator case. At Women's

Workout World, your sweat is *your* problem, but here they clearly take care of you.

"This is *way* fancy," I tell Caitlyn.

"Isn't this great?" she says.

Upstairs there are more machines, a weight room, and a row of treadmills and elliptical trainers with little personal televisions mounted on the wall next to each one. *TVs*—they don't have them at my gym, I think, because the facility is too small and they'd never be able to manage the noise level with the aerobics classes or take the time to fix them when people broke them or turned the Spanish closed captioning on somehow, or stole the remotes, but I've always preferred to think that they eschew TVs on purpose, out of some kind of conscientious, Luddite principle of cardio-purity. So the treadmill TVs strike me as terribly decadent when I first see them but I get used to them soon enough when I figure out I can watch *The Daily Show.*

When I'm done I find Caitlyn over in the weights area, where she is over by the mirror doing stretches. She says she's doing the weight exercises from *Shape* magazine.

"Really? The actual magazine?" I see a copy on the floor by the free weights. She picks it up and hands it to me.

"See, I'll bring the magazine in and show it to the staff and get feedback over whether I'm doing them right," she says.

The magazine is open to *Arms & Shoulders: 15 Moves With Results,* a spread with thumbnail photos of a woman in a sports bra top and Capri pants. Most of the photos show her from the side, a small dumbbell in each hand, elbows bent carefully, lunging and flexing in neat, hiero-glyphic poses.

"Ooh, I like her outfit," I point out. "Those pants."

"They tell you where you can get the clothes," Caitlyn says.

I do some of the bicep curls with her. I watch what she does and then I watch the mirror. It's very slow. I feel like one of those methodical animatronic dolls that people put in their windows at Christmas. I lift my handweight instead of an electric candle.

"I'm not good at this," I tell her.

"You don't have to be *good*," she says.

"I know." Though I think maybe what I mean is that I'm not good at taking it seriously.

After our workout Caitlyn convinces me to get this peanut butter protein smoothie at the juice bar. It tastes like a Dairy Queen Blizzard in an alternate reality. Maybe I could get used to this.

Caitlyn says she wants to start doing a weight loss diary online. "Just sort of on the side, apart from my regular web-site. I just really want to make an effort now."

"How much do you need to lose?" I look at her and guess. "Twenty-five or thirty pounds, maybe?"

"I was down almost fifty right after college," she says, "but this time I want to do it right, you know?"

I look around. "This seems like the place to do it." It's nicer than my apartment. I wonder if I should join when my Women's Workout World membership runs out. Working out here would most definitely be a step into the realm of Doing It Right, doing it thoughtfully, even. The people here don't seem to be the twitchy, compulsive step-aerobic drones that I see at my gym sometimes; here, in the warm coffeehouse glow of the oak floors, the people seem sociable and enlightened.

"I know," says Caitlyn. "They really go out of their way to be different. Like you," she says.

"You think? I don't know. Maybe I'll join. It's way more than I can afford, though."

"They have specials," says Caitlyn. "And you deserve it. Really, you do."

Caitlyn, I've noticed, likes to make proclamations like that. And I think I like to hear them, too.

"So does it really help to do the website?" she asks. "To write about your progress?"

"Oh, it's hell." I laugh. "There'll be people out there who are going to be in your business. Some are going to write you with all kinds of weird advice, and then others are going to think you're this expert and ask these nutty questions that you have no idea how to answer."

"Questions like what?"

"Like how many calories it takes to lose a pound," I tell her.

"Thirty-five hundred, right?" she says. "Oh, I know *that*."

screws

For weeks now my scale has had trouble staying calibrated. The needle is always half an inch or so below the zero line, making it about five pounds off. To fix it I have to turn a little metal knob at the side. Except now the knob's been turned so many times over the months it's flush up against the side of the scale and it almost can't be turned any more. I've had to get down on the floor and turn it with all my might. It's exactly like turning a screw that's all the way in already. And now, once I manage to adjust it, I weigh myself and then the needle returns, defiantly, to its place at negative five pounds, as if adhering to the laws of some parallel universe where there's ever so slightly less gravity.

I'm thinking there's got to be a way to reset the knob or something. If I can take off the bottom panel and open up the scale, I think I can pull out the threaded rod that the knob turns on. And then, well, do something with it.

*   *   *

Suddenly, it's almost spring; it's uncharacteristically hot out—muggy and warm, and I feel strange without my big coat. I've just gotten through two weeks of deadlines at work. One night I dreamt I was swimming and somehow washed up on the outdoor patio of this bar I'd gone to with Nathan once, a place where I thought, *This will be nice in the summer when we go here.* In the dream everyone was wearing skimpy summer clothes—sundresses with thin little straps; camisoles; sandals. My jeans and sweater dripped water all over the patio while everyone stared, and I wanted to run back into the lake but I couldn't find which way the beach was.

The other day I posted an entry about how I haven't worked enough, and I've been eating crappy food, and I feel bad—*bad* is the word I used, though I suppose I meant to say that I felt sluggish and sort of lost.

Two hours later, I got an email from a reader who's written me before, a woman named Paula. The subject line read **sigh . . .** and the email went:

> *I hadn't read you in a while (busy!) so I dropped by today. I have had such hopes for you and your message of body acceptance but I have to shake my head when you say you feel "bad." Because, honey, I am so, SO tired of hearing girls say that about themselves: BAD. Right now it sounds like you're letting your life depend on whether you've had a GOOD day and ate a tiny little salad! Sweetie, I thought you were smarter than that. I hope you find your way back to being a voice of reason. All best, Paula.*

I hit REPLY and write a great many things before deleting them all. Instead I type: "I'm sorry that I can't write the kind of things you would like me to write at this time."

When I turn over the scale I see eight Phillips-head screws. Four come out easily. Three are really kind of a bitch: I have to really press down with the screwdriver to get them to turn, and the screw heads are getting stripped.

There is one last screw that won't budge, though. I keep working on it, though, since I've gotten this far.

I got this email, too:

> Hi I have been doing WW for about 2 months now and I have only lost about 5-7 lbs. I swear I drink all the water but I don't know what I'm doing wrong. I am trying so hard because I am just sick of it and I can't fit into any of my clothes and I don't want anyone to look at me & I just want to know what I'm doing wrong.

I don't know what, if anything, to tell her; I might not even write her back. Sometimes I don't answer emails like this; I let them sit in my inbox for weeks. I am beginning to cultivate little patches of negligence. At the same time it has somehow become very important that my scale not mistake me for someone five pounds lighter.

The little X on top of this last screw is becoming a scraped-out hole because I keep gouging at it with the screwdriver. It's a little tiny pit and the screwdriver turns free in it without anything to hold on to.

Really, if I were to write her back I would tell her that Doing Wrong is the natural state of things. Just by going through my days I am Doing Wrong and in this humidity it seems to take all my effort to do otherwise, to undo. To put back in place. I'm living in receipts and envelopes and laundry and manuscripts; everything keeps getting disorganized and mislaid, and I don't know where these five pounds go either. With every turn of the screwdriver I'm trying to pull myself in or back to where everything is aligned.

I am sweating and pissed off and I keep giving up and then going back to try again. I try just pulling the back open a little bit. Maybe that last screw will pop out or else I can get at the pieces inside without taking off the back panel. Goddammit; I'll have to get a new scale anyway. I pry and bang and tug. The worse it gets the more I hope something will just happen to make it all worth it. The screwdriver catches on some kind of notch inside and I push it and something gives and then I push it again and it skitters and goes in deeper and gets stuck and I have to yank it out and I hope something happens. And then what happens is that the whole thing stops working altogether because it breaks. I've broken it.

I'm still on the floor and I scoot back and shove it with my foot. Not hard enough. I want to break it some more. I can't believe I broke my scale to begin with. *I broke my scale.* If I broke my scale in a fit of frustration and mounting rage, then it has to mean that I'm in some kind of stupid Fat Person Movie and *that* brings on even more rage.

I was trying to fix the damn thing and suddenly I'm slap-stick, I'm hilarity, I'm Dom Fucking DeLuise shaking the room.

Finally I get up and go over and just stomp on the scale. And then I start crying. I make big hooting sobs and don't care if the people upstairs hear me.

For about five minutes I cry because I am convinced my life stinks and then I cry a little longer because I realize it doesn't really stink and I'm crying because evidently I'm the kind of person who cries over stupid things. I loved that scale: I loved its clinical look, all white enamel like a bedpan. I loved that I paid only five dollars for it at a lesbian garage sale, back when the needle used to go up past the 230 mark. The scale's been where I've been and now I feel a little lost.

I pick up the scale and put it out by the garbage can on my back porch. I turn on my window fan. The emptied-out feeling that comes after crying like a goon feels good. I get the Swiffer and push it around the floor; I pick the screws out of the pile of dusty hair and plant leaves and toss them in the wastebasket. I get a big glass of water with ice and drink it quickly and fill it again. My limbs feel loose, like they've been taken off and then put back on right.

While I do the dishes I make a new mix tape to play when I go to the gym. I play my favorite songs twice; once to tape each one, and then once just to hear it play out and give way to the next song.

hardworking silence

"I just did something," Michael says. "And you might be really glad I did it or you might be mad, and I hope you won't be mad but I'll understand if you are."

This does not sound good. And he's called me at 7:30 A.M. to say this.

"What? What did you do?"

"I just really liked that last thing you wrote on your site, and so I showed it to this one editor at work," he said. He works for a university press. "This editor who used to work for HarperCollins."

"Uh, yeah?"

"And actually, I told her to look at the rest of the site, too."

"And?" I asked.

"And now she wants to show your site to an agent she knows."

"An agent for *what*?" I ask. I'm not really awake yet. I'm under the impression that the I.R.S. is reading my website for some reason.

These days when I see Elizabeth we have a little ritual at the start of every appointment where we check each other's outfits out.

"I like that top. That surplice style looks really good on you."

"Thanks. Don't you have one sort of like this? I think I saw it on you before and liked it." I sit down on the couch and she takes her chair. "Ooh, I didn't see your boots."

"These? They're just from Nordstrom Rack," she says, taking out her folder where she keeps her notes.

"I want to get new ones," I tell her. "I was looking at Marshalls the other day. I think I have to tell my mom about my website and I don't know if I'm ready to do it, and it wouldn't be a big deal except for the fact that I've kept it from her and my dad for this long. And the reason I would even have to tell them in the first place is that someone thinks it could be a book. And I don't know what to think about that. Because I didn't think I wanted to write a book. I just wanted to lose fifty pounds, which I can't even do. I totally ate a shitload of pasta this week."

"Do you want to write the book?" Elizabeth asks me.

"I don't know."

"Do you want to wait until you know for sure before you tell your mom?"

I think about it.

*   *   *

"You seem like you want to tell me something," my mom says, and then waits for me to answer.

Since my mom is a therapist, I sometimes use Elizabeth as a dress rehearsal for big-deal stuff I have to discuss, since the sound of her silence is very much like my mom's—a very hardworking silence. But I'm doing it cold this time. Cold and on the phone.

"Yeah, okay, so I might be writing a book," I tell her, and then, of course, she wants to know what it's about.

"See, there's this thing I did," I say. I hope that will suffice.

"All right," she says. "Do you want to tell me about it?" This is one of her Jedi therapist tricks, too.

"I've been doing this website."

"You mean the funny TV thing," she says. "I saw that, though you were swearing a lot."

"No, this is something different."

"So someone wants you to do a book about this," she says, once I've told her about the website. I knew she wouldn't be fazed at the idea of me putting up bad fat karaoke pictures of myself and telling the world, not when she gets to hear heroin addicts confess to turning tricks in her job. "What kind of book?"

"A funny book, I guess? I think they want me to do funny stories about *me*, and my *diet*, and life, and stuff."

"Oh, sort of like Erma Bombeck or something?" Mom says.

"Well, *no*." Though of course that's exactly how I made it sound.

"Hmm!" my mom is saying. "I can really see you doing something like that. And other people are already reading this? This is already out there somewhere?" she asks. Any moment now she could ask why I didn't tell her about it before.

"Right, but here's the thing."

"Yes?"

"I wrote about you once. Well, I think maybe twice."

I'd written about looking through the family photos with her last year, about trying to piece her together—put together this whole history of her body. I'd written about her surgeries and about how she'd gotten sick from them sometimes.

"So what did you say?" she asks, gently.

"Just that you were fat," I tell her. "Or I mean, that you are. And for a while you weren't, and then you were again," I add. "And sometimes you threw up a lot and it was scary."

I don't know whether her silence is an Elizabeth kind of silence.

The downstairs bathroom in our house was yellow; it had yellow-gold vinyl wallpaper in a dizzying "contemporary" pattern and the ceiling sloped sharply from the stairway above it. It had no windows and a droning exhaust fan. For about two years after her surgeries my mom had to spend a lot of time in there after dinner whenever she ate too much, or ate the wrong things that got stuck, or both. I could always hear her throwing up, despite the fan.

When I read a *Seventeen* article about bulimia I approached my mom and asked her if that's what she had. I was pretty sure she didn't have it, but I had to ask her. I wanted things to be different and the magazine article presented an opportunity for a shy little intervention on my part, even if it wasn't for quite the right thing.

"Oh, honey, no," she said. "It's maybe a little like that, but I don't have any control over it. I forget sometimes that I can't eat so much, and when I do, my stomach fights back." She told me not to worry too much about it.

The only part of the house where I could really avoid hearing her be sick was upstairs, in my room especially. But I had to go up the stairs right over the bathroom in order to get there. So I developed a routine where after dinner I would run up the stairs with my hands pressed over my ears to avoid hearing her ruin food. It made me furious sometimes.

"I guess I've always wondered how you felt about all that," she says. "That was such a strange time."

"I've wanted to tell you," I say.

She isn't saying anything again.

"I mean, I always wanted to tell you that, but I wanted to tell you about the website, too." I add.

"You know, you haven't even told me the address yet," she says, finally. "You *are* going to let me see the damn thing, right?" She's laughing a little.

"Oh, yeah. Right." I spell out the address for her.

"So what else is new?" she asks. "Any dates these days?"

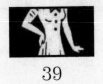

taking it personally

I am: *a woman*. Seeking: *a man*.

Age: between 25 and 42 years old. But then forty-two sounds arbritrary so I change it to forty.

It is taking me forever to fill out my profile on the on-line personals network.

Height between 5'8" and 7'0". It only goes up to seven feet. Truthfully, my experience with seven-foot-tall men is pretty limited. My high school boyfriend's cousin was that tall; I met him at a family wedding, where, later, I had to go get him for help when my boyfriend was doubled over puking in the alley behind the reception hall. The guy was easy enough to find, so why not put *seven feet* at the high end of my search range? At the low end I put my own height.

For the weight range I select *no preference* at first but I go back and change it so that the minimum is 200 pounds.

Then I'm supposed to enter a maximum and I think about it and go with *no preference* again. Guy pounds are strange. I think it's best to be agnostic about numbers.

The personality questions are hard and I answer almost all of them twice. I seem to have at least two kinds of scientific approaches here. The first school of thought is that He's Out There—or, really, *They're* Out There, since I don't like to put my faith in a fated *one*; I prefer to think that there's a small population roaming around, and one is likely to be wandering close enough by. When I list the last books I've read and the music that gets me "in the mood," I can't help but conjure up the *Whoever* who would appreciate *Kavalier & Clay*, and Antonio Jobim. And *This American Life*, and old-school Beastie Boys, and whatever other things that I think might begin to form the outline of Whoever and make it shimmer. It should be like the transport beam in *Star Trek* in that if I type in the right coordinates, maybe he'll materialize.

But at other turns the whole process seems anything but precise. I feel like I have to cast far and wide, that my ad is a radar and any half-assed garbled signal will do.

When one of my first responses comes from a guy who says: "Im easygoing and fun and I dont hold back when it comes to the joy's in life," I study the message carefully, analyzing it for alternate signs of intelligence that will cancel out the goofy apostrophes.

It occurs to me that I ought to be answering these questions under the same conditions I'd be on during a date, so one night I drink three Miller Lites before I log on. Under *Why you should get to know me*, I say, "I can put my fist in my mouth." For *Celebrity I resemble the most,* I write, "Hello Kitty." For *Five things I can't live without,* I put down "my teeth."

I show my ad to Dana when we're chatting on Instant Message one night. "Is it okay? I need feedback."

"Nice fat-girl tuck in the photo," she types back.

"Fat-girl *what?*"

"The way you hold your chin down so that your face looks as skinny as possible."

"Wow. I guess I do it without thinking."

"I do it. Everyone does it. Everyone who is FATTER IN PERSON, that is," says Dana.

Every night for nearly a week I browse the ads and steep myself in Guyness. I have lots of conversations in my head.

Dear "Sardonic_6": According to your profile, you're seeking a woman between 5'2" and 6'2" and between 110 and 195 pounds. Please advise as to whether your specifications allow for a hundred and ninety-five pound woman of any height or if a height coordinate of 6'2" is required.

Dear "NewKarma": You claim you're a "sensual idealist," but what the hell does that mean? On second thought, don't answer.

Dear Guy With A Picture Of The School Bus Driver From *The Simpsons* In His Ad: I applaud your candor in choosing to reveal your snarky prankster soul so early in our relationship. You could have chosen to show me simply *what you look like,* but then I never would have gotten to experience that certain pop-cult self-referential spirit in you which is so rare a quality among men in their twenties and early thirties. Clearly, Guy, you're nothing like Guy With A Picture Of Snoop Dogg or even Guy With A Picture Of That One *Star Wars* Character With The Ass Face. No, you set yourself apart right away.

Dear "ChiGuy": Your specs call for a woman who can be as tall as 6'3" but can only weigh up to 125 pounds. Do you have any idea what that looks like? You might want to consult the size chart on the back of a pantyhose package. Borrow one from "Sardonic_6."

Dear Anyone Who Describes Himself as a "Renaissance Man": No.

Dear Mr. No Pants: Your fellow deep-sea-diving enthusiasts may disagree with me, but I feel your reasons for putting up a photo of yourself wearing nothing but a neoprene shirt and a Speedo are just a little disingenuous. Also: "solipsism" is *not* a religion. Also: *Ew.*

Dear Every Other Guy On Here: why is "that one scene in *Betty Blue*" the default answer to the *Favorite On-screen Sex-Scene* question? Can't you think of anything else? Because isn't the title character in *Betty Blue* completely nuts? Doesn't she set fires and poke eyes out and stuff?

Dear "WhirledPeas": Sweetie, your punctuation makes you sound like you own a four-foot bong. There really is such a thing as too many ellipses.

Be real, says one of the clever taglines that goes with each profile. Clicking on *Get Matched* brings up a whole list of them, with their thumbnail photos and catchy one-line statements. I don't know what it means that there are an awful lot of pithy philosophical slogans about reality: *The only word that should always be in quotes*, and *Reality isn't as boring as we are told to see*, and *Life is surreal*, and *What is real?*, and *Reality is for losers*.

It's the same thing with the word "normal," I notice. *Why be normal? Normal is boring.*

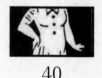

last nerve

For about a month now I have been at the business of meeting and not meeting the Nerve ad guys. I have two general rules, which is that it's usually better to meet them 1) as soon as possible and 2) only if they have a picture.

I've also learned that claiming that I can put my fist in my mouth is a very bad idea. It seems men don't think "cute, quirky party trick" when it comes to that sort of thing.

I've encountered two different guys who claim to be working on screenplays, and they're both named Eric. I met Eric #1 for coffee and General Rule #2 was born. I told Eric number #2 about Pound and sent him a link. The fact that I never heard back from him after that has made me consider a possible General Rule #3: Either don't mention my website at all, or else wait until after I meet them.

I've also learned that saying I have my own website can

be somewhat akin to bragging I can put my fist in my mouth. Some guys get a sort of Porn Reflex Reaction, a look of extreme interest that fades steadily as I tell them about my online journal—my *body issues* online journal, my virtual granny panties.

"Jules" (my mind supplies the quote marks) doesn't have a photo but I'm meeting him in record time of only about eighteen hours after he first answered my ad. I was hoping that the right and the wrong will cancel each other out, but we hate each other on sight.

"Yeah, I'm Jules," he mumbles, when I find him at the bar.

He is too pasty for *me* to be too fat for *him* but I'm sure he'd disagree. I can tell he thinks I am too dippy for him to be too hoary and weird with his black shirt that's either misbuttoned or unbuttoned too far. He has a drink already, so I order a beer and sit next to him.

The mutual discomfort is strong enough that I can almost hear it hum, malevolently, like a downed power wire.

"So," he says after I've settled in, "you're a children's book editor."

"Uh, yeah."

I am trying to remember when I told him this. In the course of three short emails, I don't think I ever mentioned it.

"So is that interesting?" he asks. He doesn't make it sound like a terribly probing question.

"It's all right," I say.

How does he know? I say in my ad I am a writer/editor. His ad says he's "a musician and chaser of demons."

"Yeah," I continue. "Um, picture books . . . mostly." I never gave him my last name. He would have to know that. He couldn't know that. Maybe I told him on the phone?

"Wait," I say. "Did you look me up on Google?"

He doesn't say anything.

"You got my name off Caller ID. And then you looked me up? Right?"

"Yeah. I did." He looks a little irritated. He explains that he just likes to "find things out first."

"One time I looked up someone and found out she used to be a man," he says, so clearly he feels there is a cautionary lesson in all this.

"Well, I'm not a man. Most women aren't."

Really, I'm pissed because I would've appreciated a chance to Google him, too, but all I had was his creepy, uninspiring first name. He wouldn't have found Poundy.com, since my full name isn't anywhere on the site, though I sort of wish he had. I get the sense that in his book, being overweight ranks just slightly above gender reassignment in terms of deal-breakers.

Everyone does this, right? Everyone looks up their dates on the Internet as soon as they get the chance. Not everyone uses what they find as a presumptuous icebreaker, but still.

"So if *I* were to look you up, what would I find?" I ask him.

"I don't know. Not much, I don't think," he says.

"Well, I mean, what do you do? You said you're a musician?"

234 · *I'm Not the New Me*

"I write and produce things," he says.

Every time he says something he sips his drink, and every time he sips his drink he shuts up.

"Okay. So what are you working on?"

"A rock opera."

"A rock opera?"

"I've just finished it." He sips his drink.

"You mean you wrote it?"

"Yes."

"Wow, a rock opera."

"Yes."

A rock opera. Who writes a rock opera? Who does this?

"What's it about?" I ask him.

"Hmm," he says, as if this is a question he doesn't much like to answer.

Who writes a rock opera and then casually mentions he's written a rock opera and then sits back and stares off silently into the middle distance? Who the hell shows up on a blind date and says, "I've written a rock opera," and expects that to just *settle the matter* and be the final and authorative word on the subject of What The Fuck Do You Do, Mr. Guy Who Just Cyberstalked Me? Who wears open shirts like that, like a male figure skater? *Who?*

"I mean . . ." I search around for another way to ask him. "Just—what's the story?"

He sips his drink and looks around the bar.

"It's based on *Othello*," he says.

"Okay."

"But modern."

"Wow. What's it called?"

"Othello."

"Okay."

He turns back to his drink. I drink mine as fast as I can.

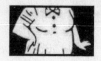
delaware

This one is insistent. The tone of his emails is, *Look, here, me,* which would annoy me but for the way they seek only my attention. He says he's writing only me.

He says he was going through the Nerve ads to make fun of them until he came across mine. "I mean I've been looking at it for a month now," he says in his first email, "and it cracks me up every time."

His name is Matt. He comes to Chicago every other weekend to visit his six-year-old daughter, Meredith—"the funniest person I know," he says. He lived in the city for years but now he lives three hours away in Madison, where he's doing some kind of database consulting for the university. He grew up in Delaware. For some reason this thrills me: *Delaware!* I didn't know people actually came from that state. He used to study film and screenwriting in college. He's thirty-six.

While I wait for him to write back I look at his profile some more. Last great book he read: *Frog & Toad Are Friends*—"It's all been downhill since then," he wrote. In his bedroom one will find: "Nothing without a search warrant."

There isn't a picture. "I'm trying to find one," he said in his first email. "I really didn't set out to put up a profile but I needed one so I could answer yours."

His next email:

> *What haunted me after sending that last email was that I left out something that, for me, nearly goes without saying: that I want to know more about you. That I'm incredibly interested. I think that you'll manage to witness me be silent like few ever have, as I listen with complete absorption. That sounds cheesy. But seriously.*
>
> *Here's what I want to do: Yes, meet up soon. Definitely. Yes, call, at the very least.*

Matt has an NPR voice on his voice mail message. Or maybe a PRI Public Radio International voice. Whatever: Matt sounds like he knows the difference between those. His voice is like the voices I get all crushed out on while listening to the public radio shows on WBEZ—guys who are not just smart but bright, funny, and a little goofy, and bristling with nervous energy; guys with their shit together, who buy decent sheets once in a while; you could even say nice sheets—sheets they may actually get a little excited about in spite of themselves just because they, the sheets, have such tangible good quality to them and they, the *men*, might think for just a moment about how buying these sheets might represent a sort of turning point in their lives and their priorities, but only for a moment, because, all things considered, guys are guys. I leave a message Sunday afternoon and two hours later he calls me back.

"Hang on," he says, early into the conversation. I hear him put his cell phone aside; he's talking gently to someone, saying, "No, you can't talk to her today." He's using a Daddy voice.

"Sorry," he says. "That was Meredith. She likes the name Wendy. She's very jealous that I get to talk to a Wendy."

We'd meant to call each other just to set up a date but we wind up talking for nearly two hours, until the phone receiver feels hot against my ear and I'm pacing around. He tells me he flunked out of college once and I tell him I've been on Weight Watchers. He has been amicably divorced for two years. "I wish I didn't live so far from Meredith," he says. But he had to take this job in Madison; it was the best offer he'd had since his last job was eliminated.

"But it's good you get to see her so often, though, right?" I tell him. He says he sees her every other week.

"Yeah, but kids at that age need beatings at least *once a week*," he says.

"Oh yeah?" I'm laughing.

"I'm thinking this probably isn't the sort of thing I should joke about with someone I barely know, is it?" he says.

"It's all right," I tell him.

"But maybe I won't always barely know you," he says.

We keep talking for another hour after that. The whole afternoon is a wave that curls over us.

In the picture he sends, he looks like a young dad; like one of those guys I see in my neighborhood; they're out on the sidewalk in front of their houses when I walk by; they smile and shrug affably while nearby someone little nudges along on a tricycle. These guys and their families almost always disappear to the suburbs by the time the kids get to school age, which makes them very mysterious to me. I imagine Matt carrying his little girl on his shoulders. And I mean, I like kids.

I don't mention the website, though I almost tell him about it at least twice.

His next email says,

> *So, let me say that I loved our conversation. That I told people about it. That you continue to impress the hell out of me.*

During another phone call he says, "You have just have such a way with words. Just . . . so funny."

"What, in my emails?"

"Well, yeah. And like now, when we're talking. God. I have to come to Chicago this week."

"You sure do, sir."

I don't tend to think that he's a hundred and fifty miles

away. More like he's *just* out of sight; just around the other
side of some door or wall or corner I'm about to turn.

Wednesday night, he says, in his next email. Can he
come up then? Wednesday is on the other side of us for
what seems like the longest time.

This is too easy for me. I live only two blocks from the
place where we're meeting. We're supposed to meet at nine
and at seven I call him.

"All right, so you know how we're meeting at Bransfield's?"

"Sure. Is that still okay?"

"Yeah, but I want to make sure you know it's the *new*
Bransfield's. The one by the Jewel on Lincoln and Cullom.
It used to be further up on Lincoln but it moved, or I mean,
it closed and reopened over here, and the place where it
used to be *still* looks *exactly* like Bransfield's, like so much
like the old Bransfield's still that I think sometimes people
who don't know that Bransfield's moved still go to that
place and *think* it's Bransfield's but just with a different
name," I say.

"It's all good. I know where to go."

"I just don't want you to wind up at the wrong place.
At, like, a phantom Bransfield's in a parallel universe."

"It's not going to happen," he says. "If I don't find the
real world Bransfield's the first time around I swear I'll keep
looking."

"Good. I'm just nervous."

"I'll see you and you'll see me," he assures me. "And
we'll be in the right place."

*   *   *

"What are you reading?" He's come right up to me at the bar.

I show him the weekly paper I'd picked up by the door and I say normal things and not, *HEY, WAIT IT'S YOU*.

He says, "Let's get a table," and I want to say just, *Hi*. I want to say, *Are you Matt?* I feel like I'm about twenty seconds behind but I'm thinking it's okay, it's fine, he's here already, and it's him.

"So, have you done this before?" he asks. "This ad thing?"

"Sure," I tell him.

He confesses that this is his first time doing the personals. "I don't know if I even *want* to be doing them," he says. "I mean, though this—here—is different."

"Oh, yeah?"

"I just felt like I really had to meet you," he said.

His eyes are distracting. They are pool blue and they pretty much knock me down. He has a ruddy, Irish face and I want to grab the sides of it.

We talk about the personals and strange pickup situations. He says he's been hit on by two women at the playground where he takes his daughter. I tell him the story of Rock Opera Guy. He has a story about getting drunk on a date and trying to make a shortcut through an alley and being chased by a giant rat (*chased*, he insists). I tell him about a blind date I had once where the guy showed up stoned and somehow talked me into going back to his tiny studio to meet his pet rabbits, who scooted around in his kitchen while I watched him play Quake on his computer.

"This date is going a little better, right?" Matt asks. "Because I've got Doom Two and you can watch me play *that*."

"So I have this website," I tell him, and I watch for the Porn Reflex Reaction. He doesn't do it.

"So tell me about it," he says.

This is the part I'm never good at.

I tell him that it's a journal, which is like a weblog, except not, and does he know what a weblog is? Because it, my site, is *sort of* like that, but the stuff I write is longer. I have to upload it all on my own instead of using something like Blogger, which I can explain if he's not familiar with it, though really, I just mentioned it because everyone keeps asking me about Blogger these days. "Anyway, my site, it's about how I lost weight last year, but I'm trying not to make it a diet journal, because I hate that, so really, it's about how I hate that stuff, and yeah. And I guess other people read it," I say. Wow, listen to me: it's All You Can Blather Night at the word-salad bar.

"And are you going to tell me the address?"

"Oh. Sure." I find a pen and write *poundy.com* on the back of a receipt I've found in my bag. "Check it out." I give it to him.

He holds the slip of paper and grins. "So this is you," he says.

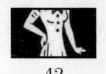

happier

It's four in the morning and there's no reason why I shouldn't stay up. I'll watch the sky get brighter and I'll get dressed and go to work two and a half hours early. Matt left at one and I think he's still driving, and I can't bring myself to sleep while he's making the trip back. If I sleep I'll disrupt the current of whatever it is that just happened.

I need to stay up and think and then I need to go to work.

I never see the intersections this quiet. I should eat something but I don't. The buildings in the office park where I work appear bigger when the lots are empty. I worry that the first things I notice after last night will be the wrong things somehow; as if I've been given a new spirit only to go out and break it with ordinary things.

* * *

It's only ten to seven but his email is waiting for me. He says there was an accident on the Kennedy on his way out; it took him forever to find an open on-ramp; he says he got pulled over an hour later and got off with a warning. Then, after that, I-39 was closed, fifty miles south of Madison, and the detour felt like the same stretch of road looped over and over, like in old movies, like where Cary Grant or someone is randomly moving the steering wheel back and forth while the background rushes past on its own. He says that none of that matters, and when are we going to see each other again.

Then, almost every morning when I wake up, there's an email from him.

He says he finds himself looking for any reason to mention me to someone, to repeat something I said. He says he rereads my emails a few too many times. We talk every night; we call and call back and leave each other long, loopy voice mails.

We keep going in the giddiest circles around each other. We start with where it started in the restaurant and then we remember everything after that: when he came up the next weekend and we went to find some place to get dinner and he stopped me on the sidewalk so we could kiss; I took a day off and took the train to Milwaukee to meet him; we got Indian food one night and he played an old tape of himelf playing really bad guitar that he'd recorded in tenth grade. We go back over everything and follow it forward and we keep stumbling upon the present where we're happy; each time we get happier.

* * *

One by one I tell my friends about him. When I tell Leigh she puts down her drink and comes across the table and hugs me.

I sign him up for my email notify list so he'll know whenever my site is updated. "I don't need this," he says. "I go to your site every day."

He lives in a nearly empty apartment in a duplex on a quiet street in Madison. It's two stories with lots of stairs, a few pieces of new furniture, and piles of CDs . He has pictures of Meredith all over; I can't get enough of looking at them because she looks so much like him.

We almost don't go anywhere when I'm there. The first afternoon we hurry through the rain to get lunch at a little deli; that night we pick up pizza and bring it back and eat it while he tries to teach me a flight simulator game on his PlayStation. I watch him make blurry landscapes pitch gently away from the cockpit window. "I can't stop playing this," he says. We sit close together on the couch for the true airline experience.

Sunday morning we get on his computer and go through the Nerve personals for fun. I show him the profiles of a couple of my bad dates and for Mr. No Pants. He shows me a profile for someone named "Ambyrr," who says "Maybe, I'm Amazed" is a song that gets her in the mood and also claims to live in an English cottage.

"In *Indiana*," Matt points out. "And I don't think that is all her real hair either. But she updates her ad all the time. It's like a train wreck."

I want to know if it's true he's never written to or heard from anyone else on the personals.

"You can see right here," he says, and he clicks on his account to show me his messages: they're all either to or from me. "Here's where it all started."

The messages are all from April; the very first one was from April 4. I'd written him back the next day.

I look at the calendar above his desk. Today is April 27.

"Can we just lie back down awhile?" I ask him. I sit on the floor and he climbs out of his desk chair to be next to me.

"Let's lie down here," he says. I let myself fall back onto the carpet; it runs up all the stairs and through every room. It occurs to me I never hear our footsteps here. I lie back and lift my arm and he lifts his and twines it around mine.

I can feel the strength in his arm, and all these little bristles in the carpet give an oddly uplifting sensation; I feel borne up. I say, "I love you," just the way we've been saying it for days now.

found

The static on Matt's cell phone sounds like the road or like a wind he keeps disappearing into.

"I'm just past Rockford now," he says, which means he's well on his way. He will likely call again when he hits Hoffman Estates, about an hour away. He'll tell me if he's making good time and usually he is. We've been doing this for five weeks now.

"You know, I'm fine with this distance thing," I'd told him. I imagined there'd occasionally be some weeks where we wouldn't get to see each other at all.

"Nope," said Matt. "Not if I can help it." He says he is going to see me as much as he can and he does. He has been coming over twice a week, sometimes coming out from the suburbs where he visits his daughter. He stays as late as he can before driving the three hours back.

This must be what we do when we're serious.

Sometimes when he's not around I almost wonder if I just made him up, especially since he's the kind of person I *would* make up; very much like the guy I'd put together from all my best impressions of grown-up guys other women get to marry. Guys with vague coolness in their pasts, like a band (Matt was in one) or film degree (ditto); who buy houses and nice things unconspicuously; be snickeringly funny; be articulate; tidy in that really cute dad-packs-for-a-business-trip kind of way. And Matt is pretty much all of those things.

"I think I thought about you before I met you," he says. "I mean, like years ago. Does that makes sense?"

"Oh, definitely."

"Sometimes I think maybe you found Poundy.com before we met in person," I tell him one night over the phone.

"Really?" he says. "Why do you think that?"

"I don't know. Just looking back." Something about the way he was that first night. I have this itch in my head about it. If he'd wanted to find me he could have; he's smart enough.

"Interesting," he says. "You think I looked you up or something?"

"Sometimes I think you did," I say. "You *did*, didn't you?"

I don't hear anything on his end for a moment.

"If you'll remember," he says carefully, "when you told me about your site I'd said, 'Are *you* going to tell me the address?' I never said I *hadn't* seen it."

"Oh, you are so busted, dude." I'm triumphant. I'm going to call him Stalker for days.

"So I didn't lie. I made sure never to say anything that would be a lie in case you ever figured this out."

"I knew it. I knew you would try."

He'd put my email address into a search engine; he found my user profile for a bulletin board I joined a year ago, then he searched on the screen name I used there— Wendola—and found my staff credit on the Television Without Pity site, which links to Poundy.com. At one point, he says, he'd stopped and wondered if he shouldn't be doing this. When he found Pound he was going to ask me about it when we met in person.

"But then you were telling me about that date with that rock opera guy, and I couldn't."

"It's not really the same thing," I insist. "It's not like you were looking for anything bad, right? Except—what were you looking for, exactly?"

"That's what I've been trying to figure out." He says after the first time we talked he had this idea that there was more to me somehow. He said I'd practically hinted.

I remember I said, "There's a little more to me than what that picture shows," but I was talking about my weight. I point this out to Matt.

"That's what you think," he says. "I think you were hiding and you wanted to be found."

"Well, then you did, I guess. And you read it?"

"I read everything," he says.

*   *   *

I'd bought a pack of cigarettes and smoked almost half of them one night, just at home, until I remembered that I've come to hate chain-smoking.

"I guess I was trying to fill myself up somehow," I tell Elizabeth. Only I don't know why I didn't just eat or something.

"So you feel—what, empty?" she asks.

I think about it. "No. It's different. More like I was trying to fill myself *in*."

I haven't written anything on my site in weeks. I've been so happy I've all but vanished there.

"I don't know if I should mention you on Pound," I tell him. I was thinking of giving him the nickname "The Professor."

"Why not?" he asks.

After Nathan I'm more cautious; when I finally mentioned we'd broken up I bristled at some of the emails I got. Some were from people simply asking me what happened and I didn't feel up to explaining; others tried to give me awkward and not always relevant advice. A couple seemed to offer the verbal equivalent of a hug with gentle hair stroking, and then there was one from "Aeon Flux" where she blathered some crap about self-love and healing. But then at the same time I was touched by everyone's concern; touched and guilty feeling because I felt like I let everyone down.

I explain that people get a little confused sometimes and they think what happens to me is just a story, even though they understand, on a basic level, that it's real.

"Do whatever you want," says Matt. "I think most people are smarter than that, though."

"You think?"

"I do. But maybe you should think about what you want, too."

Sometimes he calls me all throughout the drive home to Madison, even though I feel better hearing when he's actually *physically* home, and out of his car, his damn Jetta Turbo that he drives with a police radar detector. Until then, he's a voice cutting out.

"I'm going to update my site tonight, finally," I tell him during his last call from the road.

"Good. I'm going to sleep as soon as I get in," he says. He never stops to nap. He drives straight through and then sleeps.

While he's sleeping I write a very long journal entry. I write about meeting him, and about distance, and how it's strange that the thing that makes him the most real is the distance, or the fact that he keeps crossing it. I don't give his real name but I point out, just for kicks, that the letters in it are made up entirely of straight lines so it wouldn't be too much trouble at all to carve them into my forearm. It might creep out some people, but Matt will know I'm kidding and he'll think it's funny.

I write to tell everyone what's happening and to say, in so many words, that I'm back, or that I'm trying to get back and I'm bringing him with me.

Nobody's met him yet but this is the next best thing. Anyway, this is where he found me in the first place.

I put it up on my site the next morning. I send out an email to my notify list and I hold my breath. Within about ten minutes I get about half a dozen replies. I hope one is from him but they're all from regular readers: one from a woman who says she felt the exact same way I did when she met her husband; three are from people who have just written short "Wow!" or "That's great!" messages; and one is from Lexy, who says, "OH MY GOD! That was beautiful! What did he say when he read that?"

Oh, good question. A few more emails trickle in but none from him.

"Just wanted to see if everything's okay," I say in an email to him. "Maybe you've just been away from your desk this morning. Or maybe you don't know what to say."

He doesn't write back for an hour and I nearly curl up and die.

"I feel so lucky," his email begins. "Thank you. I have so much more to say than this. I love you. Thank you."

We are seeing Fritz Lang's *Metropolis* accompanied by a live orchestra at the old movie palace in Madison. We're in the balcony, perched high up. The theater is full, the seats around us are packed. We're together in such a tight space, our knees pressed together, but then all around us is the enormous vault of the movie theater; the intricate ceiling and the great big proscenium. We're squeezed in next to each other and we're on the edge of everything else.

The lights go out and the movie starts and the orchestra starts in. The overture races along. He has my hand;

he's letting me grip it. He is always in my head and my ears, always in the close quarters of us talking on the phone, or writing each other, or hearing each other's messages. But now here we are facing a screen, and the music is booming and startling and happening to us.

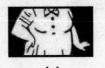

nice try

"I think I'm going to do this," Caitlyn says. "It's in June.
Check it out." We're checking our emails on the comput-
ers at Cheetah; I joined last month after my Women's
Workout World membership expired.

Caitlyn clicks on a link in one of her emails. The page
that comes up is a site for a women's triathlon.

"It's actually sort of a special triathlon," she says. "It's
for people who are new to the whole thing and who
aren't necessarily athletes." She scrolls down and clicks
though a couple of the pages to show me. The whole
thing appears to be named for and sponsored by a
women's sportswear company. "Join other women in an
experience like no other," reads the bold type at the top
of one page.

"Wow, well, it looks cool," I say, looking over at her
screen. There are words like *strength, power, confidence, joy,*

set in elegant fonts as part of the site design. It certainly looks like they have their shit together.

Caitlyn closes her browser. "Yeah, I'm probably going to register for it." She gets up and grabs her gym bag. "Hey," she says, "you should do it with me."

"Really? Oh, I don't know. I've never really done anything like that before."

I think, people always say that in movies: *Well, gosh, I've never done anything like that,* and then there's a quick cut or a fade out and then the next thing you know they've got the bungee harness on, or the motorcycle helmet, or they're topless and whooping and flinging mud, having clearly given themselves over to their true natures and doing exactly whatever it is they've never done. I wonder what it means that I am thinking this. "You should," Caitlyn says. "Just think about it?"

"I will. It's probably still pretty hard, though, huh?"

"I've heard it is, but they have this whole training schedule that you can follow. They sort of lead you through everything. They make it doable, you know?"

"Doable, yeah." We are walking down the street to our cars. Why did I drive? I bet I could get a bike and ride here.

"I'll send you the link to that site. I think you have until the end of the month to register. Seriously—consider it," Caitlyn says. "It would be awesome if you did it, too."

That night she sends me the link to the triathlon website. "Be sure to look at the training program stuff," she writes.

The site has photos of women of all different sizes and

ages, running and biking and swimming. The pictures are gorgeous and compelling. I see a photo of a woman with a number scrawled in marker on her taut arm, which strikes me as cool and vaguely kinky.

I go to a page called *Get Ready! Get Set!* There is a big pink calendar that follows three months of training, with dates marked for events like Bike Basics and Swim Clinic. They have phone coaching, email coaching, support teams. It looks like when you do this you *do* this, and I could, I think; I'd *have* to do it, and the fact that I'm even thinking this is surely a twinge of *my* true nature.

I get a little overwhelmed clicking on the calendar days: all this time stretching ahead in little squares like spaces in a board game. I could follow it until the day where I'd hop off the last space, only of course I wouldn't *hop* off; I'd run off, and swim and bike off—or, you know, in whatever order you're supposed to do it in—and people would cheer for me and I'd have a number on my arm, and I'd be beautiful, right?

I read the testimonials from people who have done the triathlon. *When I saw the photos from the 2000 triathlon I was truly inspired to do it in 2001*, says one. So I go look at the photos some more, at women grinning and glowing, or wincing from effort, caught in midstride or midstroke with water drops suspended in the air. If I did the triathlon, I could be a part of all this beauty and claim it—all this strength and power and confidence and joy. Those words could be about me, they could precede me; it would be just like having a very tasteful, award-winning commercial for myself.

No, it would be more than that. It would have to be. I
hate how I think sometimes.

"Should I do a triathlon?" I ask Matt over the phone.

"Sure," he says.

"But it would be a lot of work, right?"

"It's a *triathlon*. Why do you want to do it?"

"Well, it's a triathlon," I say. "It's a big deal and people
do it because it helps them, you know, believe in themselves and . . . stuff."

"Listen to you," he laughs. "You don't want to do it."

"But maybe I do. You shouldn't discourage me."

"I'm not. If you want to do it you should. I'll support
you and everything."

"Are you sure? It's three months away," I tell him. It's
longer than we've been together. I think of calendar days
as things we ought to be racking up, like savings interest.

Already everything is so different. The other day he'd
handed his cell phone to Meredith so she could talk to me.
They'd gone to the Disney store.

"We went to the Mickey store," she'd told me. She
sounded younger than I ever imagined myself sounding at
age six.

"Yay, Mickey!" I said. I sounded even younger.

"Were you ready for that?" Matt asked me, once he'd
taken the phone back.

I didn't answer. "Wow, she sounds so cool," I said.

*The Woman who starts the Race is not the same Woman who
finishes the Race*, it says at the top of every page on the

triathlon website. They don't say who the quote is attrib-
uted to, but I consider it every day for about a week, mostly
out of mild annoyance.

Either I can't imagine myself as the Woman who starts
the Race, or else maybe I'm not intrigued enough by the
Woman who finishes the Race, and what's with this capi-
talized Woman anyway—is that supposed to be like the
Every Woman in that Chaka Khan song? What if I'm
None of the Above Woman, and what if it's *not* in me?

I hit REPLY on an email from Caitlyn; the subject line is
Triathlon? Last chance to sign up!

"You go ahead," I write. "Sorry. Good luck!" I'm not the
same Woman.

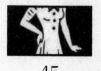

45

off

Matt hadn't mentioned coming down to see me today but he calls to say he's on the road.

"So I'll see you, what, around two then?" It's eleven-thirty now.

"Actually, it'll be just about half an hour," he says. "I'm already past Cumberland."

It feels even sooner than that. The sound of the door buzzer makes me jump.

"You're here!" I call out as soon as he's at the top of the stairs. I kiss him hello. For three days I'd been in Ohio for a children's book conference. He'd left me long voice mails and, once, we talked when I was in my hotel room and he was driving home from seeing his daughter. But I'm back and he's here.

"I have things for you," I tell him. I'd bought him stuff

on my trip—a T-shirt and books for Meredith. He comes inside.

"Can we talk about something first?" he says. He's taking off his jacket and sitting down on the bed, which is pretty much the only place to sit in my apartment. He laughs. "This is one of those conversations where you hate having to *say* 'Can we talk?' " He sits back against the wall and pats the spot next to him. I sit down.

"I'm just really, really tired right now," he says.

I nod.

"I mean, it's gotten so that it's really a problem."

I expected this. I'd expected we'd have to slow down a little sooner or later.

"You know, you don't have to drive up twice a week. I can drive up there sometimes."

"It's not just the driving," he says.

"It's not?"

"I've been doing a lot of thinking the past couple of days," he tells me. "Look, I love you, but I can't be your boyfriend anymore."

"Oh." I love him, too. He is speaking matter-of-factly, agreeably, even, enough to keep me from fully understanding.

"I'm just so sorry," he says.

He can't be my boyfriend. This might mean he just *can't be my boyfriend*. Maybe he simply *can't* the way someone can't come to a party; he will be there in spirit. He loves me, after all. He can be some kind of honorary boyfriend or boyfriend emeritus perhaps.

"I just . . . I can't do this. I really need to be a father

right now. I didn't want to come to this decision but yesterday I decided it."

I am trying to catch up with him again. "You *decided*?"

"Yes," he says.

"You mean we can't even talk about it?"

We can't even talk about it.

I can cry, though, and with a terrible rush to my head I start.

And I say, "But I wrote about you on my website."

And I hear how that sounds. So then I just keep crying.

"That's good," Matt says, his voice even and calm. "It's good to cry. I wish I could cry like that."

It's me I'm just calling I know you're probably not even home yet but I'll go on rambling here, he'd said. My voice mail system keeps bringing up old messages. I keep having to decide whether to delete or archive them. There are so many long ones. *Where are you?* He had a thing for leaving them before he went to sleep on the nights I was out. There's a lot of *I just wanted to tell you*.

There's a recent one that he'd left while I was on my trip. *It's funny, I feel almost like I'm really talking to you and not just leaving a message. Is that weird?* he says. *Like you're just here with me in some way.* Three days later he'd driven to my place and said he couldn't be my boyfriend.

Five days after that I answer the phone and hear his voice saying fresh new words.

"I wanted to make sure you're okay."

He says he was in shock after he left my place. He says

it was a hard decision and he had to tell me as soon as possible after he made it. He couldn't bear to let things "go sour," he tells me, and for some reason I thank him for this.

Just for a laugh I ask him if he left me for Ambyrr from the personals. This cracks us both up.

"You know," Matt says. "I guess I never expected that you would respond when I first wrote you. I just really liked looking at your profile and reading your answers. The one about your teeth. I mean, it still makes me laugh."

I am listening to him and I'm sitting on the floor by the window and looking up at all the same things I've stared out at when I talk to him; as long as he's on this phone I'm talking to this same patch of sky that I always have, the world is still arranged all around it.

"And then you wrote back," he says. "I couldn't believe it and then I found your site, and you were this whole person out there."

The last thing I feel right now is *out there*. Or *whole*. I'm nowhere besides this room where I live by myself.

"Am I anything like you thought I would be?" I ask.

He takes a moment to answer. "Yes, you were," he says.

The sky patch has changed since we started talking; it's getting late.

"I guess this is it," he says. "We have to get off this phone."

"I know," I tell him.

I point out that I have this Off button on my cordless phone and somehow it's harder that way, harder than with the older phones where you'd just put the receiver gently to rest.

"Meredith has trouble with the Off button, too," Matt says. "To a kid who doesn't know how phones work it seems like any other off button—like a light switch. She's trying to understand that when you hit the button it makes the people go away and you can't undo it."

"Wow. That really is sort of a hard concept when you think about it."

"Yeah, how you can't just push it again and make them come back."

"It's beautiful," I say. "That's such a beautiful analogy." Then I start crying. "Oh, shit. I'm sorry." I can hear him clearing his throat but he doesn't say anything. "I'm sorry. I love you." I cry harder.

I cry hard enough that I can't speak anymore and I have to push the button. I push it twice and listen for him to be gone.

opening

For the first days afterwards I just wanted to shut everything down. I wanted to have a blank page and I wanted people to come and wonder what happened; I wanted him to see it; see that he'd gone and broken something, he went and ruined it for everyone; nobody gets to come and get their daily dose of Poundy.com hilarity with bonus thoughtful body-image critical theory action, thanks to Matt Weisenhauer of Madison, Wisconsin, and his irrational relationship antics. Way to go.

Taking down my website, I thought, would be on the order of shaving my head, or numbly setting an old sofa on fire, or staggering around screaming and raging in a spectacular monsoon. Only tidier. Depending on the various ways I could go about it, killing Poundy.com would be either so reversible it would be almost meaningless or else so permanent that I'd surely regret it in a way I never would a burnt-up sofa. So I did nothing.

Now Richard and Nicholas have me over to their place a lot and we watch TV on their modular couch.

"I wish Matt was on *Survivor*," I tell them one night. I've cultivated a fantasy where Matt is a reality show contestant.

"He would totally do something like that," I tell them. "I mean, he decided to just chat me up all way from another state. He probably goes out trolling for Internet dream girls all the time. Because he's nuts. Definitely nuts enough to go to some demented casting call."

If he was on a reality show it would be really validating to watch, because I'd get to see confessional interviews with the other cast members talking about what a tool he is. I am sure it would be obvious. He'd make it almost to the final elimination rounds. He'd last long enough for everyone on the Television Without Pity bulletin boards to come up with a nickname for him and refer to him in pet phrases like *crazy-as-a-shithouse Matt*. Plus he'd look good in tattered Bermuda shorts. I'd enjoy it.

"I wish we'd met him," says Nicholas.

"I do, too," I say, sadly.

"Well, I mean so that we could better visualize him getting a Guinea worm pulled out of his foot," Nicholas explains.

When I was eleven I got to appear in a community theater production of *Antigone*. My grandfather dabbled in acting and he played Tiresias, and as he was playing a blind person he needed a servant boy to guide him, a Seeing-Eye Kid, so I was recruited to play the part. I was given a tunic with a hood to hide my hair, and I was instructed to never look into the audience. "This is *Greek Tragedy*," the director explained to me more carefully than necessary, "so you don't wave at your friends, okay?" Instead, I was to stare out at the dimly lit exit doors far in the back of the junior college auditorium. I held my eyes fixed on those doors even on the night that two girls about my brother's age sat in the front row and whispered loudly behind their hands. The lights made my scalp throb and I wanted badly to meet their eyes or even mouth *shut up*.

These days whenever I write on Pound I wonder if Matt is still reading, or if his sister is. I feel like I write against the glare. I want him to see how hard it is for me in *my* Greek fucking tragedy.

At work I open a manuscript called *The Sad Little Box*. It has the following verse refrain:

> "Nobody wants me,"
> the cardboard box sighed.
> "I'm sad and I'm lonely
> and all empty inside."

You know, I think, maybe the box *should* be empty for a while and just deal with it. What does a cardboard box with low self-esteem do, anyway? Go live on the street? Inside *another* cardboard box? For Christ's sake.

One morning I go out to my car and get in and sit there

for a moment with the door open, futzing around and getting CDs together. And then something brushes past my head and thumps and flutters right next to me. I scream a short scream and flail around and jump out onto the parkway. There's a bird in my car and it can't get out.

It hurls itself against the dashboard and I watch its little bird mechanisms try to reconcile itself to the space and finally it alights on the passenger side door. By the time I make it around the car to open that door, the bird has ricocheted all around the back windows and now it's trying to find a way out through the rear windshield.

It's a small brown bird. It perches on the ledge behind the backseat. I open one of the back doors but it won't come out. I open another door.

Eventually I realize that even if I open all the doors I still won't be able to bring the concept of *open* to this fucking bird. I can't do it, I can't make it; the open air has no properties that spontaneously react with bird. The world is just strange and finally its randomness brings the bird back out.

barb and wire

I keep almost getting up to close the door to my office. I don't want to close the door before I have to, but Barb the agent is going to call me today. I almost never have any reason to close the door in my office for a phone call; I did when I made my first appointment with Elizabeth, and then once when Nathan called and I tried to talk a little, well, affectionately to him, and it was awkward, and he'd said "Um, are you drunk?" even though it was two in the afternoon.

But now, I get to close my door for glamour: Barb.

A few months ago I got a phone call at work from someone who *said* he was an agent, and was trying to get me to read a children's book manuscript, a fantasy adventure (he'd called it) about a toy koala bear who comes to life after he learns to believe in himself, and then I think there was supposed to be some message about avoiding drugs or maybe even sexual abuse. "I own the licensing rights for the name 'Kevin Koala,'" he'd said. "This is gonna be big."

I could tell the guy wasn't really an agent but was trying to impersonate one to represent himself. I think about him as I wait for Barb the Agent to call. I wonder if he ever got anywhere. It seems almost too much that I had to turn the poor guy down while I wait for my call of interest from, you know, Barb, Barb the Agent.

Barb is very nice. She sounds warm and she insists she's extremely glad to talk to me. She tells me how she used to work with the ex-HarperCollins editor, though it wasn't at HarperCollins, and then she worked for a big literary agency and then she started her own agency. Michael already told me the name of one of the books she's sold recently; even though I hadn't heard of it I looked it up on Amazon and could see that indeed it was, well, a *book*, with reviews and everything.

Barb says she's read almost everything on the site and she thinks the Frequently Asked Questions are hilarious. "I could see them in a book," she says, "like as these little quips in between sections."

"Yeah!" I say. Quips! Sure!

"I just think your whole approach is very refreshing," she says. "How you're really not trying to be perfect."

"Oh, I screw up all the time," I tell her. "Ha!"

"What I'm thinking is that this could be a diary sort of format," Barb says. "I mean, I guess you *are* doing a diary, right? Like that, but a book, with just short little bits about your progress and your setbacks, because you have to have setbacks, of course, I'm sure you do, and then, of course, some of your wisdom, your attitude."

"Would this be something different from what I'm doing online?" Meanwhile I'm trying to think of what my wisdom is.

"Well, you know how *Bridget Jones's Diary* was all about her weight, like how she lost it all and she listed her weight in almost every entry," says Barb.

"I never thought of that book as . . . a weight loss book," I tell her.

"Well, no, but it's an issue. The weight. And with the actress having to gain weight for the movie."

"Renee Zellweger?"

"It's all very interesting," Barb says.

She asks me how many diets I tried before this—before I "found something that worked."

"I don't know. None really. Like I never really made an effort before this. I just decided to do Weight Watchers because they didn't seem all that diabolical or anything, and I did what they said and stuff," I tell her.

"So . . . it's not like you went and tried a bunch of crazy things, like, you know, a bunch of fad diets or something." She sounds almost disappointed. "Like—I don't know, if you ever did anything kind of extreme, like you starve yourself, or you eat nothing but, I don't know, the cabbage soup or something, or . . ."

"Or have your mouth wired shut?" I ask, because suddenly I remember something from a long time ago.

"You had your mouth wired shut?" she asks.

"No. I sort of know someone who did, though." It was Mrs. Lacey, a woman my mom knew when I was eight or so. She'd come over and bring her kids Troy and Evan, two boys about my age, who'd have high-pitched, complicated fights in my room. I noticed something wrong with her the day she burst in and muttered furiously at them. Her face was moving bizarrely, her jaw stiff but her mouth moving, like in *Clutch Cargo* cartoons. Later my mother explained what Mrs. Lacey was doing, though I could tell from her tone of voice that she didn't think it was a very good idea. For at least a year afterward I was under the impression that people with braces were desperately trying to lose weight.

"But this isn't someone you've known recently," Barb says.

"No. Sorry."

"And it's not something that *you* would have done," she says.

"No way," I tell her. "Still, it would be kind of funny to write about."

"I'm just trying to help you figure out what the story here is," she says. "*Your* story. And I know from, well, my experience"—suddenly she sounds like she's shifting position in her chair, or kicking a shoe off, getting comfy and confidential—"I had to lose fifteen pounds last year and, like, I would pretty much try anything, you know?" She laughs a little.

I laugh, too. "Yeah. God. I was never like that." Then I realize how that must sound.

* * *

"So how much weight *have* you lost?" she asks, sort of delicately.

About 35 pounds, I tell her; I make sure to mention I started at 230 and now I'm 195.

"And you still have, maybe, some way to go . . ." She is drawing out the last part as if trying to decide whether or not she's asking a question.

"I'm trying to figure that out now," I say. I explain that I think I'm going to lose more weight but who knows if I'll get much further than this.

"You *should* try to go further," she says. "I bet you can do it."

"Yeah, but you know, there's that thing about how I'm not perfect, so if I *don't* maybe that'll be okay?"

"Well," she says. "I think we really want to keep the self-help potential here."

"Self-help?"

"I think it'll be why people will want to buy this book," she says.

"But . . ." I don't know how to say this. "I didn't imagine myself that way."

"Don't you think people are motivated by you?" she asks.

Maybe, but that's *their* problem, I think.

"How did it go?" Michael asks me.

"I don't know. Sort of strange." I tell him about Barb's idea for a quirky design where my weight could appear on the corner of every page, or every other page. "Some kind of fun format like that, you know?" she'd said.

"So are you going to talk to her again?" Michael asks.

"No," I say. "I don't think I'm really what she had in mind."

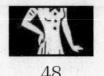

someone else is the new me

"Hang on," says Caitlyn. "I have to upload my new pictures to the site." Her boyfriend took them last night, she says. We're at her apartment after the gym.

Caitlyn's site is called *Belly To Go* and has very reliable progress photos that show her in front and back and profile, and she wears the same clothes whenever possible. When she first opens up the files and shows me, they look exactly like the first set of pictures she'd put up on her weblog; it's not until she puts them on her page that you can tell there is a change; a most distinct and empirical change. She's lost twenty pounds, thanks to her weight loss blog, or else her motivation, some of which she says she got from me.

"Oh, bullshit," I tell her. "I think it's mostly you." She's very determined. According to her weblog she's been working out at least three days a week since May, doing spinning and some weights and triathlon training stuff.

"No," she says. "You're definitely helping me."

I tried going to one of her spinning classes with her and it sort of killed me. "*Wendy* joined me in spinning class today," she'd written in her weblog, like I was making a celebrity cameo of some kind. I did feel sort of special.

"I mean, all along you've been doing this whole weight-loss thing very sensibly and with a sense of humor and I really admire that, you know?" she says.

I think, why the hell can't it help *me* lose twenty more pounds? In the past two months I've let more than five creep back on. Maybe almost ten. I have to keep making progress.

"And you don't hate yourself, either," Caitlyn is telling me. "I think you have a very high sense of self-esteem about the whole thing, and I do, too."

"Yeah, not like some people, I guess."

Caitlyn and I have been sort of tsk-tsking over a few of the other weight loss journal weblogs she's shown me. One is a girl who recently confessed she wished she had the same kind of exercise addiction a friend of hers does; she'd linked to the friend's site, also a weight loss journal, a grim little page with nine-point pale lavender type and an account of how she'd just emptied her kitchen cupboards and thrown almost everything out. The girl and the friend are 143 and 136, respectively, or so they were the last time we checked. We check again today.

"Good Lord, they're so *sad*," Caitlyn says, as we sit and read through their latest entries.

"Yeah," I say. I suppose I knew there are women like this out there. I wonder if any of the twentysomethings in the advanced step class I used to watch at Women's Workout World think this way. Sad Girl #1 is writing about how she needs an "extreme" day every now and then where she has nothing but sports shakes and vitamin-fortified water.

"I mean, I need a day every now and then where I can drink a *beer*!" says Caitlyn. She holds hers up like a trophy and I do the same.

When I do everything the way Caitlyn does the world seems a little crisper, a notch brighter: the *one* light beer after the workout tastes just cold enough and wet in the mouth and ideal; one beer and maybe one more, if I take the time to really appreciate it. There are big tall windows in the gym that look out over the fabulous neighborhood, and when I'm on the treadmill I make sure to try and look out and remember where I am, and how I make these decisions to better myself and consider all these little tangible rewards—this magazine I've bought, these little towels. Caitlyn and I talked one day about what a good idea it was to make yourself a meal by following a recipe, a *healthy* recipe, and then sit down and eat it at a *table* with a good book. I tried doing it; I mean, I *did* do it and it was nice, but I need to try doing it again and hope that after all this—after a couple weeks with Thai carryout and late nights at the Nut Hut, after Matt and after everything— that my better life will take like a graft.

You know, kids, I ate a cheeseburger the other day, writes Caitlyn in her weblog. *A BIG one*.

And it was damn good. I don't feel guilty about it one bit. That's right. Not guilty.

Because you know what? I know it wasn't a wise choice. And I am willing to accept that once in awhile I'll want to choose unwisely. As long as I understand what my body needs to be healthy.

Caitlyn has a special feature on her site that allows readers to post remarks in response to every post; you can click on a special link and a little window opens up where you can scroll through the comments:

"Yes! THANK YOU," says someone signed Carol.

"Excellent thought for today," says a Lisa M. "I'm so glad you said it."

"I agree. How refreshing."

"Caitlyn, this nearly brought tears to my eyes. I think I needed to read this today."

Some of it reads just like fan mail. I guess in a way it *is* fan mail. It's sort of like *my* fan mail, I guess, only my fan mail isn't out there for everyone to see and read in a little pop-up window in a way that might be just a little vulgar if you didn't know Caitlyn was such a sweet person. I wonder if she knows how it makes her come off. Someone should really tell her.

Every day I skim her comments page out of concern for her in this way. Really, I can't even read it. And then when I click over to Poundy.com my page feels like an empty room.

"Thank you so so much for linking to me," she says one day in the locker room. "My site stats are way up."

"Good," I tell her.

"I'm getting a lot of people writing me about the triathlon," she says. "I can't believe all these people who want me to do it."

That night I click through her comments section and see Aeon Flux has posted. "I, too, have embraced the idea of eating only fuel foods," she says.

Some of the other names seem familiar, too, now that I think about it. I think some of them were my readers. Some of these women might have been the ones who have written me and linked to me and, well, *considered me their inspiration*, even though I tend to think that's a little fucked; no, it *is* fucked, and really, I wasn't going to stand for that, and seriously, these women who considered me their inspiration really needed to go off and do something better with their time but *goddammit* that didn't mean they had to go and be all inspired by Caitlyn, who actually *does inspiring things* for fuck's sake. I click the corner of the comments window and make it vanish.

"Okay, so that weblog *Belly To Go*," I start.

"Yes?" says Ericka.

We've been chatting online for two hours now. She keeps providing a running commentary of the movie *Men Don't Tell* on the Lifetime Network. *Judith Light's feathered hair in this scene*, she'd just typed, *makes me happy to be alive*.

"Does that name make sense? Belly TO GO? Doesn't it sound like instead she WANTS a belly? And that she's going to order it at KFC?"

"Oh, Caitlyn?"

"*Where,* incidentally, she says she still goes sometimes, only she is sure to take off the skin but she'll *have the biscuit* because *by God she's a regular gal.*"

"Is she the one who's doing the marathon?"

"TRIATHLON," I type. "She will *not* shut up about it. And I know when she does it she's going to give this huge big total Oscar speech thanking the 500 people who supported her and blah BLAH."

"So she has a cheering section," says Ericka. "It probably helps her."

"And seriously," I say, "does she think there's a special club she's going to get into for being so *smart* about it? Like a Mensa for your ass?"

"You know, all that stuff's not really you anyway," says Ericka. "And you know that."

"I know." I just feel strange. I thought I knew what I was doing, that I wasn't letting myself get too caught up in trying to lose another five pounds. It's one thing to think everyone else has it wrong but it's another to see someone doing it more right than I will ever manage. I keep looking at Caitlyn's page, where she's written about some fancy expensive cross-training shoes she's bought; she's included a picture of herself holding them up and smiling in amazement.

"Wendy, she is kicking ASS right now. Kicking it HARD," Ericka types.

"I know, okay? And I guess I can't stand it. There's a part of me that wishes I was where she is."

"What?"

"Caitlyn."

"No, JUDITH LIGHT is kicking ass," Ericka writes.

"Oh, in the movie?" I grab the TV remote.

"This is the one where she BEATS her husband! Ha! She is TOTALLY WHALING ON HIM NOW!"

"It's just that it makes me feel like I have to lose twenty more pounds to be sure of what I'm saying," I tell Elizabeth. "And then I know that's stupid, so I want to *gain* twenty pounds just to show how stupid that is."

The theme of today's session with Elizabeth is I'm Jealous And It's Okay, and I do most of the talking, as usual.

#

because you have to have setbacks of course

I am eating bread. It's what I eat when I eat too much. I mean, behold the gory details of my excess: *bread*.

I know what everyone is saying about carbs these days, but it still feels like eating enough bread to gain weight is pretty pathetic—it's like getting addicted to Robitussin or spending your life savings on Lotto tickets. For Christ's sake, prisoners in dungeons can barely stay alive on the stuff, so how in the hell is it making me fat?

Lately I have a thing for incidental bread, like hamburger and hot dog buns. Eating a hot dog bun by itself is like getting by on a technicality; really, what's being consumed is less "bread" than it is "absence of hot dog"; it doesn't count because I'm eating the inessential part of the sandwich. A couple times I've found myself tearing off pieces of plain flour tortillas, which extends the logic a little too far, but then again I guess I must be so desperate that the food sort of wouldn't count either; I'm hungry in a way that doesn't need to be filled so much as cancelled out.

i just called to say

There was no Lite beer at the motherfucking German-American fest; I've been trying to be good but fun conspires against me. Fun and Rolling Rock in a plastic stein that was bigger than I thought.

I was with Leigh, and Leigh's a bartender, and I was trying to keep up with her, and probably I shouldn't do that, should I? I decided that it would be the best thing to come home.

We ran into Stuart tonight, of all people. He was making his way through the crowd with a couple of Leigh's other bar regulars and a date much closer to his age and height. We all stood around shouting over the noise of the people and the oompah band. Stuart struck me as ingratiating and a little smirky. "How are *you*?" he said.

"I'm fine!" I'd shouted. All the Bavarian cheer was making me feel thuggish. I bopped him on the arm. "How are YOU?"

Fine, he'd said. "Great!" I said, giving him a jolly shove.

It was getting dark and the crowd outside the main tent was getting denser. I was feeling restless. I hit Stuart again. "Howya *doing*?!" I said.

Leigh gave me a look. I turned to her. "I know it's bad to hit the little man," I said. "I'm sorry." I turned back to hit Stuart. "Howya DOING?!" I screeched.

It was time to go home.

I need to call Matt. He should appreciate that it's been months, like two months since I talked to him. It's been long enough. I believe he will understand that if it weren't for the fact that I am drunk I would probably not even be calling him at all, and thus I hope he recognizes that the sloshy vulnerability I am revealing to him this evening is a rare treat. A gift, even. Plus, it's only 9 something P.M. A drunk dial, I reason, can't be all that bad if I'm doing it during prime time.

There is an easy way to call him and a hard way. The easy way is on my cell phone, because his number is still stored in my phone book there; all I need to do is highlight it and select the Dial command. The other way involves my regular cordless phone, where I'd have to look at the phone number itself and take each digit and press the corresponding key on the phone and do so in the proper order without skipping or repeating any digits unnecessarily, and moreover I'd have to actually *find* the number, and the only place I have it now is on my cell phone, I think, hence the easy way.

I press my cell phone against my head until I can tell that he's answered. "It's Wendy," I call out. "Hi!"

I can just make out that he says *hi* but that's only because it's simple and the most likely thing he would say. The phone feels as useless as holding a shoehorn to my head.

"I can't hear you," I say to the phone and hang up.

I amaze myself by carefully reading his number—long distance—from the little digital display on my cell phone and dial it up on my much bigger and far more phonelike home phone.

"What are you doing?" says Matt. I can hear him now.

"Okay, this is better. I'm drunk dialing you," I say.

"Great."

I don't really remember all of the conversation even as it's happening. At one point I am telling him everything I think about what happened between us. "Like maybe you *thought* you wanted a relationship," I say, "but you didn't. You wanted, like, some *unavailable* chick, who was all *not there*, so you could *not* have a relationship."

"I'm not talking to you like this," I can hear him say.

His voice sounds two degrees removed somehow; it sounds like if it's not coming from him but from a TV or a radio on somewhere in his apartment. I try to listen to Matt talking but my attention seems to keep wandering to the background noise, to this distant call-in show with the ranting, irritable host, until I realize it's Matt's voice and Matt is talking to me.

"What?" I say.

"I'm seeing someone else now. You can't call me like this."

"You're not."

"Yes, I am."

Everything is falling away. "But you weren't going to be seeing anyone else," I protest.

"Well, you know, I guess I am," he says.

Then I am sputtering at him now, and weeping, and calling him a "fuckerhead." I ask him if he got back with his ex-wife. I ask him, with all seriousness, if it's Ambyrr from the personals. I believe he tells me it's neither of those but I'm sobbing too hard to really listen, and I am calling him a "liar shit."

"Two months!" I say. I hear myself saying that for some reason.

"No, *four* months," he says.

"*Two* months!" I repeat.

I think we're arguing about the amount of time we've been broken up, but I can't be sure, because I know it's been longer than two months. Has it been four?

I hear myself screaming, "Fuck you, Matt! *Fuck off!*"

This is not going as well as I thought it would.

"I'm hanging up the phone now," he is saying. "I'm about to end this call."

"No," I say. "I'm going to hang up first. I'm doing it. I'll do it." Somehow I do.

not butter

I know the phones have something to do with why I'm up
so early. My cell phone is on my nightstand and my cordless phone is on the mattress and it's as disquieting as waking up next to a couple of grenades. I move them but I
can't go back to sleep because now I remember.

I don't think I have a headache, but I don't know if I
even moved all night; I feel like I slept pressed under a
board laden with bricks.

I feel mostly leaden except for a thudding sense of
shame that becomes worse the longer I'm awake. It gets as
lucid and real as he's suddenly become again; after all these
weeks he'd become indistinct enough for me to play
around with the idea of him; I'd made up various versions
of him, sweet and stoically heartbroken ones that turned
out to be all wrong. Everything becomes worse the more I
remember for real.

I must have passed out before eleven last night; it's eight now—not a good 8 A.M. either, with clear sunlight. The sky is just gray-white and stopped up; it feels like anything that might help me right now is inextricably stuck behind it.

You're up early, Ericka types. Nobody else is online except her.

"I know." I guess I shouldn't be surprised that she is on. She is on a lot; she lives in my computer, I think.

"Time for your fancy new gym?" she asks.

I just type *no* and close the window.

Sometimes people go away if you stop answering them. Or they'll stay online but they stop typing messages and it's like they're gone. She won't mind; she'll let me be off somewhere busy.

But a new little window pops up and in it she says, *Something's wrong, I think. Yes?*

"I drunk-dialed Matt last night," I tell her.

"The Professor?"

"His name is Matt." I wish I never gave him that nickname. "He's just some guy who dated me by mistake."

"Oh no," she says. *Oh no,* she keeps typing as I tell her about last night.

"So how do you feel right now?" she asks.

Like my head is all stuffed up with something; like there's a big wad of cotton or lint that is dulling everything and I'm trying to dislodge it with hamburger buns, empty hamburger buns spritzed with *I Can't Believe It's Not Butter!* spray.

"It is like a sandwich," I tell Ericka, "made of emptiness and disbelief. Literally. I mean, practically."

Go on, she types out.

"I was trying to make a joke about the sandwich."

"I know. But go on," she tells me.

"I don't know what to do. I want to just disappear," I write. "I mean sometimes I do. And I don't mean like dying or anything."

"You don't have to mean it that way for me to listen," she says.

It's almost ten and I ate the rest of the buns. It's still overcast outside; I'm all full of starch and so is the weather somehow.

"I'm trying to think of things that will make you feel better," Ericka is typing.

"Thanks," I tell her. "I think I'm okay." It helps to talk.

"Hey, I could send you my Weight Watchers magnets," she offers.

"You mean the ones you got after you lost twenty-five and fifty pounds?" I ask her.

"Sure. And then my bookmarks, too. The I Lost Five Pounds thingies."

"Why would you give me those?" I ask her.

"I don't know," she says. "I mean, I'm kidding. I know you don't really want them."

"So I guess I could borrow them and pretend I lost a whole bunch of weight or something?" Ericka is strange.

"Sure! Why not?" says Ericka. "I mean, I wonder if

maybe you're not writing as much lately because you don't have *that* to say. You haven't been doing the diet thing as much and you think people only want to hear that."

She could be right. I stopped going to Weight Watchers about a month ago. I don't know why I decided to stop, except that I wanted some time to myself. Or else I wanted some time away from myself. I'm really not sure.

"Well, I couldn't just say I lost like a hundred pounds. It wouldn't be true."

"So what? There are lots of other things that are true," she says. "And you used to write about those more."

It's true, I did.

"Hello?" she says. I haven't typed anything for a couple minutes. I have been pulling up the edge of my T-shirt to wipe my nose and eyes.

"Okay, so why haven't I met you in person?" I ask her. "I mean, you've lost one hundred and twenty-five pounds, for Christ's sake." We always keep saying we'll meet up, but it's a long drive, and she's got a little kid, and I've got my life. "How do you lose one hundred and twenty-five pounds and then stay stuck in my computer?"

"Yeah, well, I showed you my pictures, since you were wanting to see."

"I know." She'd sent two: the first is of a woman in a nightgown; she looks about my age, short, thick hair; she's holding her daughter. I could tell it was a *before* picture from the thickness of her arm as it hooks around the baby. She is wide in her robe, but her arm looks so much like my mom's. In the second she's much thinner; she's at the zoo; she's anyone; she's Ericka. But then she's only words, too.

I think that's what gets me: after all the things a person can do to her body by running and lifting and eating and abstaining, after all that work she can still amount to almost nothing but words. Nothing much besides a voice—a voice that gets more and more familiar—and all I can do is listen.

"And anyway," says Ericka. "I think I've gained twenty pounds back. Maybe more."

"That's okay," I tell her. I know she's somewhere out there.

which truth

The house where I grew up had a full third-floor attic. In the daytime there was always enough light from the gabled windows to rummage around, and often I'd go up to the attic for no good reason, only a vague imperative to *find* something.

I was always retrieving things of my own that I'd banished from my room at some point or another—the set of *Little House* books, rescued one at a time; old board games; a pocket radio. It seemed like I was never done with anything and I was vaguely ashamed that my bedroom wasn't big enough to hold all the things I needed. But I could never put anything completely away.

I also couldn't stay out of my mother's clothes. They were in a very large cardboard box that had once held a Kenmore air conditioner. My mom used it to store all the clothes that didn't fit her but were too good to throw out or give away; I believe there were things that were both too big and too small for her. The smallest things were size 12–14.

The first items were sanctioned: there was a dressy ruffled blouse she gave me when I was in sixth grade. "This isn't quite my style," she said. *Style* was an elusive concept but I wore the blouse at Christmas feeling grown-up and I decided that wherever my mother's style left off was where mine began.

By the time I was in junior high my style was voracious. I'd go up to the attic on my own to dig through the box looking for possibilities; for anything at all that I could wear. Nothing I owned was ever enough; my concept of what was cool or at the very least acceptable to wear changed constantly. One week I'd want to dress like Kelly Ferrara, who had sweatshirts in all kinds of Starburst candy colors; the next all I'd want was to wear something unobtrusive enough to avoid the attention of Patty Melko, a eighth-grader who'd squint at me across the lunchroom whenever I wore something ambitious, like my one yellow sweater from Limited Express, and then invariably step up to interrogate me later. "Why are you so *gay* in that outfit?" she asked me once.

I went through the attic box looking for anything that was the right color for whatever I was striving towards, or the right collar; anything I could work with. The sizes didn't matter—in fact, my mom's fat clothes were serendipitous for the '80s. Almost nothing was ever too big, especially not if it was worn on top; sweater hems that went halfway to my knees were just fine with me; once or twice I made safety-pin alterations to the ankles of my mom's pants to try and simulate the baggy harem style. If I had no clear idea how to appear, I knew at least how to lose myself. And maybe lose my mom a little, too.

"It's a mess up there," my mom said more than once. "Everything in that box used to be folded. I know you're taking things."

I'm just *borrowing* them, I'd insist.

"As long as that's *all* you're doing to them," she'd say, because I'd cut the sleeves off one shirt after they'd failed to stay rolled up to my liking.

"You were ruthless," my mom says now. "You went through everything and just helped yourself. I mean, Jesus. Anything in that attic was yours as far as you were concerned."

We're in the kitchen of my parents' new house. They've lived there for ten years but it's still sort of new to me—a single-story ranch house in Willow Springs, with a big garage and a tiny crawlspace attic that can only be reached through a trap door. My dad says they were sick of paying the high property taxes in Oak Park, and anyway, my mom's knees were bad and they wanted a house where she wouldn't have to climb so many stairs.

"Yeah, I guess I really was a little shit sometimes," I say.

"Well, I think you were just being creative," my mom says. "That's the way you are."

"I guess," I say, though I think *creative* is too kind a way to put it.

My mom was never going to be a thin person, despite the surgeries, and the attic was where I learned to understand it. My mother put on weight imperceptibly enough from day to day to escape notice for a while, but in my own way I'd begun to piece together which body of hers was the truth. Or which truth I preferred.

"Why is *this* in your closet?" she asked me one morning. She held up a black knit top I'd taken. She'd burst into my room half-dressed and headed straight for the open wardrobe where she found it. I was in ninth grade and thus had developed the tendency to be unsettled by the sight of my mom's Mom Bra and its severe elastic engineering. Right below her bosom was the long, cross-hatched surgery scar that ran down the middle of her abdomen; I never really liked looking at that, either. Now she pulled the shirt off the hanger and glared at me. "*Why?*" she repeated.

I didn't have an answer. I loved the shirt for the way the collar opened sideways with silver grommet snaps, and so I'd taken it straight from her closet.

"It's like you think I don't even exist," she said, and marched out. I gave her credit for wanting it back so much.

Now my mom tends to say fond things about the way I was. "You had a style all your own," she says. I think of it differently: in my mother's clothes I didn't have to own anything about me. I had a secret, unspoken but incontrovertible excuse for whatever shortcomings, real or imagined, Patty Melko or *Young Miss* magazine or anyone else might find in me: everything was my mom's, and my mom was fat.

If I lived in this thought for years it's probably no surprise that my own body grew used to the comforts of home, so to speak.

Today is my mom's fifty-ninth birthday; we ordered Chinese food and my dad picked up an ice cream cake for the occasion. When it got late my brother had to leave to drive back to Wisconsin, but I've stayed a little longer to help my mom with the last of the cake.

"I'd have you kids take some of it with you but it would melt," she says, so we cut two wedges of mint chocolate chip and eat them out of bowls at the kitchen table.

The cat, Zipper, sits across from my mother and waits. He understands, after years of experience, that anything a family member eats from a bowl will eventually be his to lick. He also has an uncanny ability to sense the exact moment when my mother finishes, and he always saunters across the table just as she takes the last bite.

"I think he can tell by the sound of the spoon hitting the side of the dish," she says. "It must sound different when the bowl's empty."

We watch him clean the bowl and then he sits back, licking his face for as long as it takes for him to be content.

So here in the kitchen I'm telling my mom that I think I'm going back on Weight Watchers, because I guess I should, because my clothes are a little tight, like not *that* bad, but I probably shouldn't let things progress much further. And that I might put a second weblog up on Poundy.com where I write about *just* the weight stuff and not anything else so I can be focused, and also, I can tell it makes a difference when I don't go to the gym, and since it's summer I haven't really been going, and God, I'm going to have to do something, right?

And when I say all that I just might mean: *It was hard for you, so see how it's hard for me, too?*

"Oh, you look good," my mom says.

And when she says that I think she means, *Oh, you look good.*

"Well, thanks," I say. And *I'm sorry.*

And she hands me the bowls to put in the sink.

The kitchen in this house has a counter and a bank of cabinets between the breakfast nook and the rest of the kitchen, so that you can stand at the sink and talk to someone without quite being in the same room as them. "Do you feel ever weird that you gained the weight back after the surgery?" I ask. "Or I mean, how do you feel about all that?"

I know she can answer this just fine. I wouldn't have asked if she couldn't. But I also have just never asked.

And she tells me: she says she wished she hadn't, of course. She says it was good just to *do* it. There was a time she'd convinced herself that she was just too far gone, and the fact that her body had this potential to change, that despite everything it could follow the logic of science, that therefore she was still a part of the world, part of everything.

She tells me this, though of course I'm not remembering her exact words here. I mean I have to paraphrase for reasons of my own.

"I don't see why you need to add another online diary thingy to your website just for your diet stuff," my mom says.

I resist telling her that 1) everyone says *weblog* these days and 2) nobody says *diet*. These would require too much explaining, though.

"Honey, if you had a page that was just your diet stuff," my mom says, "it wouldn't sound like you."

She might be right.

"Well, maybe I'll just do this other thing I was thinking of doing, then," I say. "This thing where I'd have to borrow your scanner."

"Ask Dad," she says. "What do you want to do?"

"Remember those nasty Weight Watchers cards you had? I was thinking about putting them up on my site. With some funny commentary maybe."

"Why on Earth would you want to do that?" my mom asks.

"I don't know. They're *gross*. Just because."

"You're weird, my dear," she says.

#

amelia Earhart is my favorite athlete

Caitlyn did the triathlon. She was just as I'd expected: the Woman who started the Race and the Woman who finished it and then not the same woman as either of them and certainly not me. What I hadn't expected was how beautiful she looked in the picture she'd put up on her site—with the marker scrawls on her shoulder, grinning and glowing and completely at rest.

"*Oh, my God* I'm going to be on *Good Morning America*," she said when I returned her call. "Tomorrow. They're doing a segment on weight loss journals. I get to go down to the ABC studio and go on satellite. *Oh. My God.*"

"What time? Early, right? I'll definitely record it," I told her.

300 · I'm Not the New Me

I wouldn't admit to getting up and watching it live instead of getting ready for work.

"Lots of folks are losing weight over the Internet!" one of the teasers said. "Could it help you, too?"

The segment went well. Caitlyn is a good interviewee and she came off like an expert, which I guess she is.

I liked her much better than the doctor who went on and on about the "need to fight obesity." Then he said, "You should always use caution when you follow advice you find on the Internet." I gave him and the TV the finger.

There was a lot of interest in Caitlyn doing the triathlon. Robin Roberts asked her if there were any athletes who inspired her. "Just all the women who did the triathlon with me, Robin," she says, which is a very good answer. At the same time I realized that it's not a question I would ever, in a million years, want to be asked.

Later that day, though, an answer came to my head—Amelia Earhart, though of course she's not an athlete. But duh: neither am I.

When I drive home from work lately I go past an old industrial area that is being developed into a couple of strip malls; all this new construction with fresh white curbs. They're putting in a Panera bakery just like the one we stopped at in Ohio and down the street there's a sandwich chain that I saw in Madison when I visited Matt. It's a little weird how the signs and the logos and the shapes of the buildings make me think so specifically of the other places I've seen them, though I know that's exactly *not* the point of them.

And when I go by the newest buildings covered in Tyvek now I wonder not only about what the new places are going to be but also whether they're going to be in the *Weight Watchers Fast Food Companion*. I mean I keep thinking of how when you're on something like Weight Watchers you're not only supposed to be watchful, you're supposed to be everywhere. You have to be everywhere at once in time to stop yourself.

One day in June I'd tried to go to the gym. I hadn't gone in a couple of weeks. I stopped at the Cheetah front desk and gave my membership card to the guy there to swipe. He handed it back and I started towards the stairs to the locker room.

"Whoa. Hang on," he said, looking at his computer monitor. He held his hand up. He wore a red string bracelet just like Madonna. "You're not paid up this month."

"Really?" My membership was set up to make automatic withdrawals from my bank on the fifth of each month. I tried to remember if I had any money in my checking account on June 5. My rent check must have just barely gone through.

"Do you want to try to run it through again now?" he asked.

It was the 10th. "No," I'd said. I had a feeling things weren't much better. I didn't want him to look up my account and see for sure. "I'll pay later this week."

He made a note on my record. "You can work out today but next time you need to be paid up," he said.

"Thanks," I told him. I changed, did weights for forty minutes and left. I forgot to go back later that month. My July dues didn't clear either but by then I'd decided to wait out the summer.

I am taking walks, instead, especially when I can get to a party that way. I feel like I've slipped off the radar.

I stopped going to Weight Watchers meetings weeks and weeks ago. I have my membership booklet in the bottom of my purse. I changed purses last month but I did take a moment to put it in the bottom of my straw bag, instead of just sticking it in the desk. So it feels like I am keeping up in some manner. But then, it keeps occurring to me that maybe I can go through life and just not get fat.

I don't know when I stopped believing that my body is tugged along by some kind of destiny *toward* or *back*, or that the distance between two points in one's life is always charted as an angle: that there's a hill to knock myself out on; that my next movement will take me up or down.

The only thing is that I don't know where I am these days. I am somewhere just downwind of someone else's pot smoke. An awful lot. I'm not smoking it but I'm not moving, either, and my whole summer seems to be just like that.

The email reads:

> *Dear Wendy, I've never written you before but I just wanted to say thank you for your journal and for sharing everything the way you have. I'm saying it now because I don't think you're going to be doing it much longer. I mean*

I guess that's the feeling I get from you not writing in it as much as you used to and that's okay. Anyway, thanks. best, Jen.

I need to write her back to tell her she's wrong. Any day now I am going to write something new if that's all it takes to be right.

I could still make things simple. Any day now and I could pick the day and start there. I could find my way to straight ahead. I could plug myself in and make everything simpler and simpler; breakfast, lunch, dinner. I could repeat myself until I made myself clear. I like to think I did, like the frames in a film, moving fast enough to make the image alive.

Once I stepped on the bathroom scale at Leigh's place and what I saw was okay. So I do it again at a party, some place where we've made our way one night in early August. I find the bathroom and when I see the scale I go over and step out of my flip-flops and stand, and hear the way it *pings* only the way a stranger's scale sounds.

I look and then go out and to the kitchen, and then out to the porch where everyone is gathering in the new blue night where you can see the clouds still holding the last bit of sun. Soon it's dark enough to follow the tips of people's cigarettes. I don't even remember what I saw when I looked on the scale. I don't quite remember the numbers, though I have an idea of what they are. I keep checking to see if I'm lost but I'm not.

* * *

I park the car at Montrose Beach. I've brought a bottle of water and a book to read. As I'm crossing the park on my way to the sand my cell phone rings; it's Richard.

"I'm at the beach!" I shout. "I am all deep in thought."

The wind has picked up. "I just got here," I yell. I keep yelling. "No," I shout again. "I don't know. I just felt like it. No. FELT LIKE IT. *FELT!*"

He thought I said "fell."

The sand here is the color of old paper and is speckled with glass and shell bits. There is brilliant glint on everything, on litter and toys and wet kids. A man is throwing a ball across the distance to his dog and they keep changing positions in the deep space of the clear day.

Everything glitters except the lake, which has a blurred edge. The horizon is matte and the lake is a flat background. It's like a test pattern and I can't stop looking. The only thing that convinces me it's real are the moving airplanes, including a small one trailing a banner for a radio station.

I walk in up to my ankles and then up to my knees and then I have to stop. I am standing here in my clothes with my bag at my side and my shoes in my hand. I didn't know I'd want to swim.

I guess I wouldn't know: I came all this way in my head. I came as far as I could, just to the water.

But then the water is good and cold and wherever it hits my skin begins. It keeps insisting *here* and I believe it.

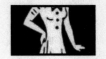

the end

Acknowledgments

Michael Taeckens anticipated this book long before I did and I can't thank him or love him enough for his encouragement, energy, and friendship, though I'll gladly run up huge long-distance phone bills while I try.

I owe so much to my agents at the Gernert Company—to Erin Hosier, for her tireless support, and to Betsy Lerner for her guidance. Thank you, Megan Lynch, for being a thoughtful editor and a reassuring presence, and many thanks to Julie Grau, Craig Burke, and everyone else at Riverhead Books.

I couldn't have finished this book without a residency at the Ragdale Foundation, nor without the support and infinite patience of Kathy Tucker and the folks at Albert Whitman & Company.

Thanks to Sarah Bunting, Tara Ariano, and the Television Without Pity staff. Thank you so much, Deb Stoller.

A great many thanks to Shylo Bisnett, Phineas X. Jones, Kristine Lewandowski, Brian Sobolak, Jeff Webber, Doug Wortel, and Claire Zulkey who read early drafts and/or were just there for me. Catherine Welsh listened to me, Gwen

Zepeda, Pamie Ribon, and Erin Shea inspired me, and Ron Slattery took me to the beach.

I'm forever grateful to everyone who became part of the story, especially Leigh, Ericka, and Dana. Thank you Weight Watchers, International, for influencing me in a way that certainly neither of us ever expected. And for not, you know, suing me.

To readers of *Pound* whose emails and links and visits over the past four years have encouraged and sustained me more than I can ever express: I love you all.

My deepest gratitude is for my family, especially my mother, who has always understood.

Wendy McClure grew up in Oak Park, Illinois, and holds an M.F.A. in poetry from the Iowa Writers' Workshop. She is the creator of the online journal *Pound* as well as the humor site *Candyboots*. A columnist for *BUST* and a founding contributor to the website *Television Without Pity*, she lives in Chicago.